Recent Results
in Cancer Research
88

Founding Editor
P. Rentchnick, Geneva

Managing Editors
Ch. Herfarth, Heidelberg · H. J. Senn, St. Gallen

Associate Editors
M. Baum, London · C. von Essen, Villingen
V. Diehl, Köln · W. Hitzig, Zürich
M. F. Rajewsky, Essen · C. Thomas, Marburg

Paediatric Oncology

Edited by William Duncan

With 28 Figures and 38 Tables

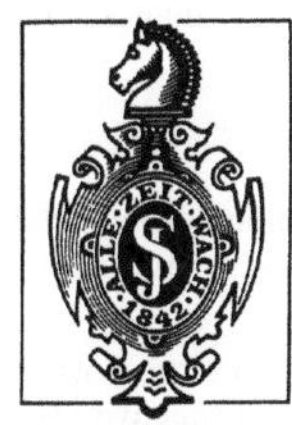

Springer-Verlag
Berlin Heidelberg New York Tokyo 1983

Professor William Duncan

Department of Clinical Oncology
Western General Hospital, Grewe Road
Edinburgh, EH4 2XU, United Kingdom

Sponsored by the Swiss League against Cancer

ISBN-13:978-3-642-82036-6   e-ISBN-13:978-3-642-82034-2
DOI: 10.1007/978-3-642-82034-2

Library of Congress Cataloging in Publication Data. Main entry under title: Paediatric oncology. (Recent results in cancer research; v. 88) Papers presented at the Fourth Symposium on Clinical Oncology held at the Royal College of Radiologists, London, in February 1982 sponsored by the Swiss League against Cancer. Bibliography: p. Includes index. 1. Tumors in children − Congresses. 2. Leukemia in children − Congresses. I. Duncan, William, 1930− . II. Symposium on Clinical Oncology (4th: 1982 : Royal College of Radiologists) III. Schweizerische Nationalliga für Krebsbekämpfung und Krebsforschung. IV. Series. [DNLM: 1. Neoplasms − In infancy and childhood − Congresses. W1 RE106P v. 88 / QZ 200 P126 1982] RC 261.R35 vol. 88 616.99′4s [618.92′994] 83-14672 [RC281.C4]

© Springer-Verlag Berlin Heidelberg 1983
Softcover reprint of the hardcover 1st edition   1983

2125/3140−5 4 3 2 1 0

This publication brings together a number of papers presented at the Fourth Symposium on Clinical Oncology held at the Royal College of Radiologists, London, in February 1982. The subject of the meeting was paediatric oncology, and its objective was to provide an up-to-date review of the management of children with leukaemia and the more common forms of childhood cancer.

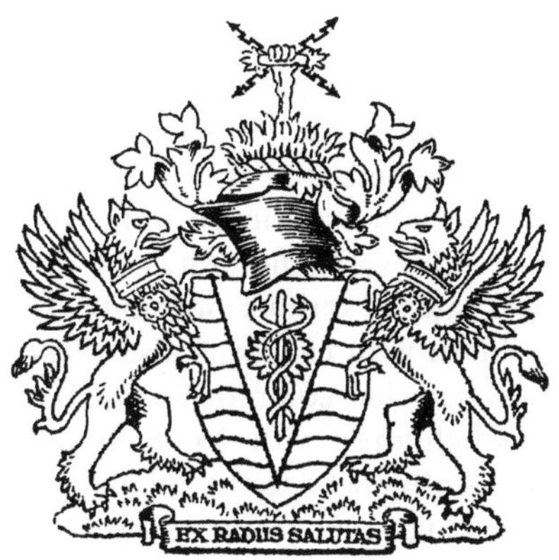

Cancer in childhood is fortunately uncommon. The descriptive statistics of these diseases in the United Kingdom, and in many other countries from which data are available, are presented in some detail. Some remarkable differences in the incidence of the leukaemias, for example, are recorded throughout the world. Further studies of the reasons for such differences hopefully may provide some insight into the causation of these diseases.

The leukaemias represent the most common form of neoplasia recorded in the Manchester Children's Tumour Registry, accounting for almost one third of all childhood cancers. Acute lymphoblastic leukaemia is the most common type of leukaemia in children in all countries for which we have adequate data, with the exception of Japan. A masterful review of the achievements in the management of acute lymphoblastic leukaemia is given by Professor R. M. Hardisty. This was his topic for the George Edelstyn Memorial Lecture which is given each year during the Symposium. The continuing improvement in the remission rates of these patients is a remarkable triumph of multi-disciplinary collaboration in management. It has also been the result of many well designed and superbly conducted randomly controlled trials. It is hoped that these symposia will encourage further collaboration, both in clinical research and in the general care of these patients.

Unfortunately increasing success in the management of leukaemia and other childhood cancer is not achieved without considerable morbidity. The psychological sequelae of childhood leukaemia are described, and the effects on parents and siblings are discussed. Constructive suggestions are made about supportive measures for the whole family during the first few months of treatment. Thereafter some families may need more specific help, but clearly further research is necessary to define the most effective intervention in these circumstances. The late physical sequelae of the treatment of children with leukaemia and other forms of cancer are also described with consideration of the improved techniques that may help to minimise or avoid these effects.

A general review is given of the pathology and natural history of childhood tumours. The management of children with tumours of the brain, lymphomas, soft tissue sarcomas, bone tumours, Wilms' tumour and neuroblastoma are in turn discussed, together with descriptions of new approaches that are being evaluated.

The best results of management undoubtedly are recorded by large groups, who, by their greater experience and concentration of special skills and expertise, achieve higher rates of remission commonly associated with lower rates of serious morbidity. This approach to the management of children with cancer is also relevant to the care of adults, particularly with the less common forms of cancer. The systemic adjuvant treatment of children with Wilms' tumour has also had an important conceptual influence on the management of many adult tumours. And so, although this group of diseases represents only a very small part of clinical oncology, the management of children's tumours is an important and fascinating subject which should be of general interest to all oncologists.

I have to express my gratitude to all those who took part in the Symposium and to their colleagues who have collaborated in writing the manuscripts which are published in this volume. I am indebted to them not only for providing the material but for their understanding in the editing of the texts in order to achieve a uniform style and format throughout the publication. I would also record my appreciation to Mr. Michael Jackson of Springer-Verlag for his support, and to Ms. Jane Teather for her expert editorial assistance. And finally I am most grateful to my personal secretary, Mrs. Joyce Young, for her constant support in the organisation of the Symposium and in the preparation of the scripts and editorial material for publication.

Royal College of Radiologists, London   William Duncan

Contents

List of Senior Authors

C. C. Bailey
Seacroft Hospital, Leeds, United Kingdom

J. M. Birch
Christie Hospital and Holt Radium Institute, Manchester,
United Kingdom

J. A. Bullimore
Bristol Radiotherapy and Oncology Centre, Bristol, United Kingdom

R. M. Hardisty
Institute of Child Health, The Hospital for Sick Children, London
United Kingdom

J. Kemshead
The Hospital for Sick Children and Institute of Child Health, London,
United Kingdom

G. P. Maguire
University Hospital of South Manchester, Manchester,
United Kingdom

J. S. Malpas
St. Bartholomew's Hospital, London, United Kingdom

H. B. Marsden
University of Manchester and Royal Manchester Children's Hospital,
Manchester, United Kingdom

P. H. Morris Jones
Royal Manchester Children's Hospital, Manchester, United Kingdom

M. G. Mott
Royal Hospital for Sick Children, Bristol, United Kingdom

D. Pearson
Christie Hospital and Holt Radium Institute, Manchester,
United Kingdom

J. Pritchard
The Hospital for Sick Children and Institute of Child Health, London,
United Kingdom

E. M. Sweet
Royal Hospital for Sick Children, Glasgow, United Kingdom

Epidemiology of Paediatric Cancer*

J. M. Birch

Department of Epidemiology and Social Research, Children's Tumor Registry, Christie Hospital and Holt Radium Institute, Withington, Manchester M20 9BX, United Kingdom

Introduction

Epidemiology can be defined as the study of the health of human communities. In looking at paediatric cancer from an epidemiological viewpoint it is important to consider its relationship to other diseases which may influence the incidence of all or some types of cancer in childhood; studying the patterns of disease within individual families may lead to discoveries of aetiological significance. In England and Wales cancer is now the most common natural cause of death in childhood and is exceeded only by accidents (Office of Population Censuses and Surveys 1978). This pattern, which is common to most developed countries, emerged in the period immediately following the Second World War. With improvements in health care and better social conditions infections, which had hitherto been the major cause of childhood death, rapidly became of less importance.

In order to plan an appropriate service to care for children with malignant disease, to provide the best possible chance of cure and to set up clinical trials of new treatment protocols, it is necessary to know the incidence and natural history of the various types of malignancy which occur in childhood. This type of information can be provided by a population-based registry. Most cancer registry data are presented in terms of the primary sites, e.g. breast, lung, bladder. This is fairly satisfactory for adult cancers, which are mainly carcinomas, but for children many of the important types of disease can present at a variety of sites, e.g. rhabdomyosarcoma and neuroblastoma. It is important, therefore, to classify childhood tumours by histology and ideally all cases reported to a paediatric cancer registry should be reviewed histologically to ensure diagnostic accuracy.

The first population-based childhood tumour registry in the United Kingdom was the Manchester Children's Tumour Registry (MCTR). It collects data on all cases of cancer in children resident in the North West Regional Health Authority area of England with child population of approximately one million. The MCTR was set up in 1954 and is described in detail by Marsden and Steward (1976) and Birch et al. (1980). Histological slides of all solid tumours are obtained by the Registry and circulated to a panel of pathologists who are expert in oncological or paediatric pathology. Slides are retained by the Registry and reviewed periodically so that diagnoses can be revised in the light of current knowledge. Ascertainment has been estimated to be 95%–98% complete (Leck et al. 1976), and the MCTR is therefore in a position to give an accurate estimate of incidence. Incidence of the main tumour groups is shown in Table 1. Leukaemias and other reticulo-endothelial tumours comprise nearly half the total number of cases. Intracranial tumours represent nearly one quarter of the total. Various embryonal tumours, e.g., Wilms' tumour,

---

* The Manchester Children's Tumour Registry is supported by Cancer Research Campaign

Table 1. Manchester children's tumour registry 1954–1980. Incidence of childhood malignant disease

	Males	Females	Total	Rate per 10^6
Leukaemia	498	389	887	32.8
Other reticulo-endothelial	200	107	307	11.3
Intracranial	326	293	619	22.9
Connective tissue tumours	150	128	278	10.3
Wilms' tumour	69	70	139	5.1
Neuroblastoma	97	71	168	6.2
Retinoblastoma	38	40	78	2.9
Germ cell tumours	24	43	67	2.5
Epithelial	32	27	59	2.2
Other rare tumours	48	38	86	3.2
Total	1,482	1,206	2,688	99.3

rhabdomyosarcoma and neuroblastoma, which occur mainly in young children and are extremely rare outside the paediatric age group, account for most of the remaining cases. Epithelial tumours frequently seen in adults are very uncommon indeed in childhood. A feature of childhood tumours which is seen in most series is the preponderance of boys among patients, especially in acute lymphoid leukaemia (ALL), lymphomas and medulloblastoma. The germ cell tumours form the only group in which an excess of female patients is seen. Incidence and the significance of these sex differences are discussed more fully in Birch et al. (1980). Details of histological features are dealt with in a later chapter.

International Variations

Until recently most data on the incidence of childhood cancer from countries other than the United Kingdom were presented by site, e.g., in Waterhouse et al. (1976) making international comparisons difficult. However, there have been a number of recent reports which classify the tumours by histology and some interesting international differences in incidence have begun to emerge.

Tables 2–5 show the incidence of childhood malignant disease in populations in the United States (Young and Miller 1975), Japan [Aichi Prefecture] (Hanawa 1975), Australia [Queensland] (McWhirter and Bacon 1981) and Sweden (Ericsson et al. 1978). Regrettably, as yet no population-based data presented by histological group are available from Africa or the Indian sub-continent.

Table 2 compares the incidence of leukaemias and lymphomas in the various populations. ALL is by far the most common type of neoplasm in all the populations except the Japanese. The figures for "other leukaemia" in the American series include unspecified acute leukaemias and unspecified lymphocytic leukaemias. These presumably would have included many cases of ALL. If this is taken into account it can be seen that Manchester has a relatively low incidence of ALL compared with the other white populations. Leukaemia tends to be an upper social class disease and socio-economic differences may account for this lower incidence in the Manchester region of England. Socio-economic differences may

Table 2. Annual incidence of chilhood malignancy in various populations per 10^6

	Leukaemia and lymphoma					
	MCTR	US white	US black	Japan	Australia	Sweden
Acute lymphoid leukaemia	25.9	24.6	12.9	12.5	31.7	29.1
Acute myeloid leukaemia	4.9	6.6	3.9	13.3	2.7	5.0
Other leukaemia	1.9	10.9	7.3	5.5	1.4	5.2
Non-Hodgkin's lymphoma	4.6	6.3	6.4	3.8	7.2	8.5
Hodgkin's disease	3.7	5.8	6.0	0.5	6.2	3.2
% Total tumours	41.4	44.4	39.1	47.4	43.6	37.1

Table 3. Annual incidence of childhood malignancy in various populations per 10^6

	Central nervous system tumours					
	MCTR	US white	US black	Japan	Australia	Sweden
Astrocytoma	8.9	8.2	8.2	1.1	9.5	14.3
Medulloblastoma	5.0	4.8	2.1	0.9	4.7	4.7
Ependymoma	2.8	1.3	1.3	0.5	2.5	4.3
Other central nervous system tumours	6.3	9.8	12.0	8.9	5.7	9.3
% Total tumours	23.0	19.2	24.4	14.8	19.8	24.3

also in part account for the low incidence of ALL in US blacks, although it is probable that ethnicity also plays a role here. One of the more interesting findings to emerge from these recent reports is the high incidence of acute myeloid leukaemia (AML) and low incidence of ALL among Japanese children. A study of childhood leukaemia in Shanghai (Li et al. 1980) indicates a similar pattern amongst Chinese children. Japanese children also show a low incidence of lymphomas. It would be interesting to study the incidence of leukaemia and lymphoma amongst migrant Japanese and Chinese in a country with large populations of these ethnic groups, e.g. the United States. This would indicate whether the differences in incidence were mainly genetic or environmental in origin and may help to clarify the aetiology of these diseases.

The incidence of central nervous system (CNS) tumours is compared in Table 3. CNS tumours, such as astrocytoma and medulloblastoma, which are commonly found amongst white populations of developed countries, are rare among Japanese children. In contrast Sweden shows a remarkably high incidence of astrocytoma. The lower incidence of medulloblastoma and ependymoma in US blacks may be accounted for by the relatively high proportion of non-specific diagnoses included in the "other CNS" group. It is possible that some of these cases were medulloblastoma or ependymoma.

Connective tissue tumour incidence is shown in Table 4. The incidence of soft tissue sarcomas is again very similar amongst the white populations of the developed countries. Although the distribution of the various types in Sweden differs from the other white populations, this may be accounted for by differences in diagnostic interpretation as the overall incidence is similar. Both US blacks and Japanese show a relatively low incidence of

Table 4. Annual incidence of childhood malignancy in various populations per 10^6

| | Connective tissue tumours | | | | | |
	MCTR	US white	US black	Japan	Australia	Sweden
Rhabdomyosarcoma	3.7	4.5	1.3	1.4	3.5	1.1
Fibrosarcoma	0.7	0.9	0	0.3	0.2	1.2
Other soft tissue sarcoma	0.5	3.0	2.6	0	0.2	2.6
Osteosarcoma	2.5	3.3	4.3	0.6	1.0	3.1
Ewing's tumour	2.0	1.7	0	0.3	3.5	1.6
% Total tumours	9.8	10.8	8.9	2.9	7.7	6.8

Table 5. Annual incidence of childhood malignancy in various populations per 10^6

| | Embryonal and other rare tumours | | | | | |
	MCTR	US white	US black	Japan	Australia	Sweden
Wilms' tumour	5.1	7.6	7.7	3.7	7.2	8.4
Neuroblastoma	6.2	9.4	6.9	7.3	8.7	6.5
Retinoblastoma	2.9	3.4	3.0	5.0	5.0	4.1
Other rare tumours	11.3	12.5	10.6	11.5	11.9	19.9
% Total tumours	25.7	25.6	27.6	35.0	28.9	31.7

soft tissue sarcomas. Ewing's tumour does not seem to occur in black children, as indicated by the study of US black children and by data available from Africa (Williams 1975; Davies 1976), and it may be that this racial group is genetically resistant to Ewing's tumour. Amongst the remaining tumours which are compared in Table 5, one of the most interesting findings is the low incidence of Wilms' tumour in Japanese children. The incidence of Wilms' tumour is also comparatively low in Manchester. It was suggested at one time that Wilms' tumour could be used as an index cancer of childhood because it showed little international variation (Innis 1973). This is now clearly not the case. Both US white and Australian children show relatively high incidences of neuroblastoma. Retinoblastoma is more frequent in Australia and Japan.

Although reasons for these international variations in incidence are not clear at present, their study is an important element in epidemiology, as this can lead to the formulation of hypotheses on aetiology. Particularly important are studies of migrant populations, as these can indicate the relative importance of genetic and environmental factors in aetiology and result in the possible discovery of environmental carcinogens. At present the only migrant populations of children to have been studied are the US blacks and children from Queensland, Australia, whose ethnic origins derive mainly from Western Europe. The study of US blacks is as yet of limited value because of the paucity of data from Africa. For more detailed discussion of the significance of the data from Queensland, McWhirter and Bacon (1981) should be consulted. There is a great need for studies of the incidence of the various histological groups of childhood cancer in Africa and the Indian sub-continent and for migrant studies in other parts of the world.

Aetiological Factors

From epidemiological, clinical and laboratory studies knowledge of the aetiology of some cancers, e.g., carcinoma of the bronchus, is extensive. For other cancers, e.g., carcinoma of the cervix, sufficient is known to be able to isolate high risk groups and to formulate some hypotheses. For many cancers, however, very little is known and these represent a formidable challenge to the epidemiologist. Childhood cancer falls mainly into this latter category.

Aetiological factors can be thought of as intrinsic, the result of an individual's genetic constitution, or extrinsic, arising from the environment and including voluntarily ingested substances such as drugs and tobacco products. Although extrinsic and intrinsic factors will be considered separately, all cancers almost certainly derive from an interaction between the two.

Extrinsic Factors

Although a high proportion of human cancers can be attributed to environmental factors, their relevance to childhood cancer in particular has not been established. In adults, cancers developing as a consequence of exposure to an environmental carcinogen are usually epithelial in nature and often occur after a latent period of some 20—40 years. Cancers in children are rarely epithelial and frequently occur in very young children, some being congenital. The opportunity for chronic exposure and long latency therefore does not exist. However, it is possible that environmental carcinogens do have a role in the aetiology of childhood cancer.

Chemical Carcinogens. Numerous examples of human carcinogens associated with occupation have been identified and some of these were recognised before the beginning of the 20th century (Eckart 1959). Although industrial exposures do not play a direct role in the aetiology of childhood cancer, an indirect role has been suggested. Fabia and Thuy (1974) reported that children whose fathers were engaged in hydrocarbon-related occupations at the time of their birth were at a greater risk of dying from malignant disease than children with fathers in other occupations.

The results of a subsequent case-control study carried out in Finland (Hakulinen et al. 1976) did not support the hypothesis that there is an increased risk of malignancy in children of fathers in hydrocarbon-related occupations. A study was carried out in Texas (Zack et al. 1980) in which information on job histories covering the time from a year before birth to a year before diagnosis was collected for case parents and three sets of controls. No increased risk of childhood cancer associated with hydrocarbon-related occupations in either parent was found. An association between paternal occupations related to lead and Wilms' tumour was reported by Kantor et al. (1979). The study was based on data from the Connecticut tumour registry and paternal occupations were obtained from the children's birth certificates. A recent analysis of paternal occupation as recorded on death certificates of children dying from malignant disease failed to produce any strong evidence for associations between particular occupations and childhood cancer (Sanders et al. 1981). The inconsistency of these various reports may reflect differences in study design and sources of data and further, more detailed, studies may clarify whether or not parental occupation can be a risk factor in the development of childhood cancer.

If there is an association between parental occupational exposure to chemical carcinogens and cancer in children, the mechanisms involved must be related to exposure of the young child to such carcinogens introduced into the house on clothing, or exposure in utero via the placenta. Other potentially important sources of transplacental carcinogens are drug-taking and dietary and smoking habits during pregnancy.

Two examples of human transplacental carcinogens have been demonstrated. Herbst et al. (1977) have shown an increased incidence of clear cell adenocarcinoma of the cervix or vagina in the daughters of women who were treated with large doses of diethylstilboestrol in early pregnancy to prevent miscarriage. Diphenylhydantoin (DPH), which is suspected to be associated with increased risk of lymphoma in adults (Hoover and Fraumeni 1975), is probably also a transplacental carcinogen. At least four cases of neuroblastoma in children exposed to DPH in utero have been reported (Pendergrass and Hanson 1976; Sherman and Roizen 1976; Seeler et al. 1979; Allen et al. 1980). Other drugs may well act as transplacental carcinogens and careful assessment of all drug exposures during pregnancy is needed.

In laboratory animals the most potent transplacental carcinogens are among the N-alkylnitrosamines and nitrosamides, and an individual carcinogen may be considerably more potent in the foetus than in the adult (Tomatis and Mohr 1973). A low dose which is not capable of producing tumours in the adult can be carcinogenic in the foetus. Nitroso-compounds occur in many foods, in urban air and in cigarette smoke (Walker et al. 1976). They may also be synthesised endogenously from nitrite and amines or amides present in food and drugs. This process occurs throughout the digestive tract and may be another source of exposure (Tannenbaum 1979). The necessary nitrosation reactions can be blocked by ascorbic acid and may also be inhibited by vitamin E (Young and Newberne 1981). Although dietary factors may be of importance, the complex nature of mechanisms of carcinogenesis and the likelihood that very low doses of a combination of compounds would be involved renders the task of identifying such factors extremely difficult.

Physical Carcinogens. There is no doubt that ionising radiation is a potent carcinogen and children exposed at Hiroshima and Nagasaki developed leukaemias and solid tumours at an increased rate (Ishimaru et al. 1971; Jablon et al. 1971). Children who have received radiotherapy for benign and malignant conditions are also at an increased risk of developing further neoplastic disease (Meadows et al. 1978). An increased risk of developing malignant disease in children exposed to diagnostic radiographic procedures in utero was first reported by Stewart et al. (1956). Since then numerous studies have demonstrated similar increased risks, but whether or not the association is causative has remained a controversial issue (Mole 1974). However, less frequent use of obstetric radiography and the lower radiation doses associated with modern techniques make the problem largely academic. At present, ionising radiation cannot be considered an important aetiological factor in the majority of cases of childhood cancer.

Although asbestos has apparently not caused cancer in childhood, an instance of mesothelioma developing in the wife and daughter (at the ages of 50 and 34 respectively) of a man chronically exposed to asbestos has been reported (Li et al. 1978). The man was in the habit of taking his work clothes home. He was a smoker and developed lung cancer at the age of 60. The case of this family illustrates the need to enquire about indirect exposure to industrial carcinogens during childhood in people who develop relevant cancers at an unusually early age. Young people known to have been exposed to carcinogens (industrial or medical) as children should be particularly advised against smoking.

Viruses. The strongest evidence for an aetiological role of a virus in childhood malignant disease is the association between Epstein-Barr virus (EBV) and Burkitt's lymphoma in African children. Infection with EBV is extremely widespread among this group and a recent prospective study (de-Thé et al. 1978) carried out in the West Nile district of Uganda concluded that, although the results supported a causal association between EBV infection and Burkitt's lymphoma, other cofactors are required and "the potential oncogenicity of EBV is realised only in exceptional circumstances". These other cofactors may be related to severity of and/or age at primary infection and simultaneous episodes of malaria. Viral infections during pregnancy have been implicated in the aetiology of childhood cancer in a number of studies (Bithell et al. 1973; Adelstein and Donovan 1972). A recent analysis of data concerned with exposure to chickenpox in utero and the development of childhood cancer did not, however, support a link between these two events (Blot et al. 1980). Whether viral infections during pregnancy can result in a higher risk of developing childhood malignant disease remains an open question, but the proportion of cases which might be attributable to such infections is small.

Intrinsic Factors

Intrinsic or genetic factors are probably of greater relative importance in the development of childhood cancer than in adult cancers. The occurrence of congenital tumours, known associations with malformations, increased risk in patients with certain hereditary syndromes and the familial nature of some childhood cancers, all indicate a potentially major role for genetic factors in the aetiology of malignant disease in childhood. The genetic basis of childhood cancer is dealt with in a subsequent chapter, but some aspects are mentioned here to complete the picture of possible aetiological factors. Susceptibility to childhood cancer may be determined by the inheritance of a gene (or genes) which results in the development of a childhood cancer such as retinoblastoma. It may be influenced by the inheritance of a syndrome which predisposes to the development of malignant disease, e.g., von Recklinghausen's disease, or by inheritance of susceptibility to environmental carcinogens as in xeroderma pigmentosum (Strong 1977). Any study of the aetiology of paediatric cancer must take into account the interaction of genetic and environmental factors.

Approaches to Epidemiological Studies

A useful starting point for any epidemiological study is the population-based cancer registry, as this is the simplest means of ascertaining cases. For calculation of incidence it is clearly important that ascertainment should be as complete as possible and that some estimate of completeness should be made. Methods of ascertainment are discussed in detail by Leck et al. (1976). For other types of study complete ascertainment is not necessary but a representative sample of the total number of cases in a population, which should be as large as possible, is desirable. Single hospital series are often unsuitable because referral bias results in an unrepresentative series of cases. The exception would be a specialist hospital in which most, if not all, cases from a particular population are treated. Where possible it is important to monitor annual incidence of each tumour type. Variations in incidence with time may reflect changes in environmental carcinogens, changes in socio-economic conditions and so on, and could be a stimulus to fruitful research into aetiology. A recent analysis of MCTR data demonstrated a rise in the incidence of ALL which was particularly marked in boys and in the younger age groups (Birch et al. 1981). More detailed studies of ALL are currently under way.

The restrospective study of cancer registry, hospital and other medical records can yield useful information. Using this approach the association between Wilms' tumour and hemihypertrophy was found (Pendergrass 1976). Medical records other than the child's own case notes can also provide valuable information. An examination of the obstetric notes of mothers of children with germ cell tumours showed a high incidence of anencephaly in the stillborn siblings of these children and an association between infections during pregnancy and early onset of tumours in the offpsring (Birch et al. 1982). The disadvantage of this type of study is that often no suitable group for comparison can be found and the significance of some findings is difficult to assess. For the incidence of cancer and some major malformations there are fairly good population data available for comparison with the case group under study, but for most other factors no such population data exist. Case-control studies, in which identical sets of data are collected for patients with a particular disease and for individuals who do not have the disease (controls), overcome this problem and have proved to be a powerful tool to the epidemiologist. In the field of paediatric cancer the Oxford Survey of Childhood Cancer used this approach to demonstrate an excess risk of developing malignant disease in children exposed to X-rays during pregnancy (Bithell and Stewart 1975). The success of a case-control study depends upon the careful selection of controls. This should be done such that the controls are as representative as possible of the general population from which the study group derives and are not biased in any particular way, for example older, or from a higher socio-economic group than average. Ideally more than one control per case, selected by different methods, should be used.

Because of the rarity of childhood cancer, prospective cohort studies, in which a group of individuals is followed for a period of time and observed for whatever factor is under study, are unsuitable in this field.

Epidemiologists should always be ready to explore any unusual observations brought to their attention. It was the discovery of a small cluster of cases of vaginal adenocarcinoma in young women, which is extremely rare, which led to the initial discovery of a human transplacental carcinogen (Herbst et al. 1971).

In conclusion, the successful study of the epidemiology of childhood cancer depends upon a multidirectional approach and on cooperation between clinicians, pathologists, laboratory workers, statisticians and epidemiologists.

References

1. Adelstein AM, Donovan JW (1972) Malignant disease in children whose mothers had chickenpox, mumps, or rubella in pregnancy. Br Med J 4: 629–631
2. Allen RW Jr, Ogden B, Bentley FL, Jung AL (1980) Fetal hydantoin syndrome, neuroblastoma and hemorrhagic disease in a neonate. JAMA 244: 1464–1465
3. Birch JM, Marsden HB, Swindell R (1980) Incidence of malignant disease in childhood: 24-year review of the Manchester Children's Tumour Registry data. Br J Cancer 42: 215–223
4. Birch JM, Swindell R, Marsden HB, Morris Jones PH (1981) Childhood leukaemia in North West England 1954–1977: epidemiology, incidence and survival. Br J Cancer 43: 324–329
5. Birch JM, Marsden HB, Swindell R (1982) Pre-natal factors in the origin of germ cell tumours of childhood. Carcinogenesis 3: 75–80

6. Bithell JF, Draper GJ, Gorbach PD (1973) Association between malignant disease in children and maternal virus infections. Br Med J 1:706–708
7. Bithell JF, Stewart AM (1975) Pre-natal irradiation and childhood malignancy: a review of British data from the Oxford survey. Br J Cancer 31:271–287
8. Blot WJ, Draper G, Kinlen L, Kinnier Wilson M (1980) Childhood cancer in relation to pre-natal exposure to chickenpox. Br J Cancer 42:342–344
9. Davies JNP (1976) Some variations in childhood cancers throughout the world. In: Marsden HB, Steward JK (eds) Tumours in children, 2nd edn. Recent results in cancer research, vol 13. Springer, Berlin, pp 28–58
10. de-Thé G, Geser A, Day NE, Tukei PM, Williams EH, Beri DP, Smith PG, Dean AG, Bornkamm GW, Feorino P, Henle W (1978) Epidemiological evidence for causal relationship between Epstein-Barr virus and Burkitt's lymphoma from Ugandan prospective study. Nature 274:756–761
11. Eckart RE (1959) Industrial carcinogens. Grune and Stratton, New York London
12. Ericsson JL-E, Karnström L, Mattsson B (1978) Childhood cancer in Sweden, 1958–1974. 1. Incidence and mortality. Acta Paediatr Scand 67:425–432
13. Fabia J, Thuy TD (1974) Occupation of father at time of birth of children dying of malignant diseases. Br J Prev Soc Med 28:98
14. Hakulinen T, Salonen T, Teppo L (1976) Cancer in the offspring of fathers in hydrocarbon-related occupations. Br J Prev Soc Med 30:138–140
15. Hanawa Y (1975) All Japan Children's Cancer Registration, 1969–1973. Children's Cancer Association of Japan, Tokyo
16. Herbst AL, Ulfelder H, Poskanzer DC (1971) Adenocarcinoma of the vagina: association of maternal stilbestrol therapy with tumor appearance in young women. N Engl J Med 284:878–881
17. Herbst AL, Cole P, Colton T, Robboy SJ, Scully RE (1977) Age-incidence and risk of diethylstilbestrol-related clear cell adenocarcinoma of the vagina and cervix. Am J Obstet Gynecol 128:43–50
18. Hoover R, Fraumeni JF Jr (1975) Environmental factors: drugs. In: Fraumeni JF Jr (ed) Persons at high risk of cancer. An approach to cancer etiology and control. Academic Press, New York, pp 185–198
19. Innis MD (1973) Nephroblastoma: index cancer of childhood. Med J Aust II:322
20. Ishimaru T, Hoshino T, Ichimaru M, Okada H, Tomiyasu T, Tsuchimoto T, Yamamoto T (1971) Leukaemia in atomic bomb survivors, Hiroshima and Nagasaki, 1 October 1950–30 September 1966. Radiat Res 45:216–233
21. Jablon S, Tachikawa K, Belsky JL, Steer A (1971) Cancer in Japanese exposed as children to the atomic bombs. Lancet 1:927–932
22. Kantor AF, McCrea Curnen MG, Meigs JW, Flannery JT (1979) Occupations of fathers of patients with Wilms' tumour. J Epidemiol Community Health 33:253–256
23. Leck I, Birch JM, Marsden HB, Steward JK (1976) Methods of classifying and ascertaining children's tumours. Br J Cancer 34:69–82
24. Li FP, Lokich J, Lapey J, Neptune WB, Wilkins EW Jr (1978) Familial mesothelioma after intense asbestos exposure at home. JAMA 240:467
25. Li FP, Jin F, Tu C-t, Gao Y-t (1980) Incidence of childhood leukaemia in Shanghai. Int J Cancer 25:701–703
26. McWhirter WR, Bacon JE (1981) Incidence of childhood tumours in Queensland. Br J Cancer 44:637–642
27. Marsden HB, Steward JK (1976) (eds) Tumours in children, 2nd edn. Recent results in cancer research, vol 13. Springer, Berlin
28. Meadows AT, D'Angio GJ, Evans AE, Jaffe N, Schweisguth O, van Eys J (1978) Spontaneous and treatment-related second malignant neoplasms in children. In: Severi L (ed) Tumours of early life in man and animals. Proceedings of the VIth Perugia Quadrennial International Conference on Cancer, 30 June to 5 July 1977. Perugia Quadrennial International Conferences on Cancer, Perugia, pp 121–124

29. Mole RH (1974) Antenatal irradiation and childhood cancer: causation or coincidence? Br J Cancer 30: 199–208
30. Office of Population Censuses and Surveys (1978) Mortality statistics: childhood and maternity. Series DH3.5. HMSO, London
31. Pendergrass TW (1976) Congenital anomalies in children with Wilms' tumour: a new survey. Cancer 37: 403–409
32. Pendergrass TW, Hanson JW (1976) Fetal hydantoin syndrome and neuroblastoma. Lancet 2: 150
33. Sanders BM, White GC, Draper GJ (1981) Occupations of fathers of children dying from neoplasms. J Epidemiol Community Health 35: 245–250
34. Seeler RA, Israel JN, Royal JE, Kaye CI, Rao S, Abulaban M (1979) Ganglioneuroblastoma and fetal hydantoin-alcohol syndromes. Pediatrics 63: 524–527
35. Sherman S, Roizen N (1976) Fetal hydantoin syndrome and neuroblastoma. Lancet 2: 517
36. Stewart AM, Webb JW, Giles BD, Hewitt D (1956) Preliminary communication: malignant disease in childhood and diagnostic irradiation in utero. Lancet 2: 447
37. Strong LC (1977) Genetic considerations in pediatric oncology. In: Sutow WW, Vietti TJ, Fernbach DJ (eds) Clinical pediatric oncology. CV Mosby Company, Saint Louis, pp 16–32
38. Tannenbaum SR (1979) Endogeneous formation of nitrite and N-nitroso compounds. In: Miller EC et al. (eds) Naturally occurring carcinogens – mutagens and modulators of carcinogenesis. University Park Press, Baltimore, pp 211–220
39. Tomatis L, Mohr U (1973) (eds) Transplacental carcinogenesis. IARC Sci Publ no. 4. IARC, Lyon
40. Walker EA, Bogonski P, Griciute L (1976) Environmental N-nitroso compounds: analysis and foramtion. IARC Sci Publ no. 14. IARC, Lyon
41. Waterhouse J, Muir C, Correa P, Powell J (1976) (eds) Cancer incidence in five continents, vol III. IARC Sci Publ no. 15. IARC, Lyon
42. Williams AO (1975) Tumours of childhood in Ibadan, Nigeria. Cancer 56: 1065
43. Young JL Jr, Miller RW (1975) Incidence of malignant tumors in US children. J Pediatr 86: 254–258
44. Young VR, Newberne PM (1981) Vitamins and cancer prevention: issues and dilemmas. Cancer 47: 1226–1240
45. Zack M, Cannon S, Lloyd D, Heath CW Jr, Falletta JM, Jones B, Housworth J, Crowley S (1980) Cancer in children of parents exposed to hydrocarbon-related industries and occupations. Am J Epidemiol 111: 329–336

The Pathology and Natural History of Childhood Tumours

H. B. Marsden*

Department of Pathology, University of Manchester and Royal Manchester Children's Hospital, Manchester M27 1HA, United Kingdom

Introduction

In the past few decades cancer has become relatively more important in paediatrics due to the advances in prevention and treatment of infections. In 1970 neoplasia was the second most common cause of death between the ages of 1 and 15 years (Marsden and Steward 1976). The improvement in the results of therapy and the study of aetiological factors have shown that paediatric oncology is a particularly rewarding field. The Children's Tumour Registry in Manchester[1] (MCTR) has kept records of all cases of childhood cancer in the North West region of England since 1954 and has provided the data on which this review is based.

Leukaemia and Lymphoma

Leukaemia accounts for one third of the cases of malignant disease in childhood, this being due for the most part to acute lymphoid leukaemia (ALL). The incidence of leukaemia is shown in Table 1 with ALL as 79% of the group and 26% of the total tumours. The other types of leukaemia are much less common and acute myeloid leukaemia (5% of the total), is exceeded in incidence by neuroblastoma (6%) and equalled by Wilms' tumour, juvenile astrocytoma, medulloblastoma and non-Hodgkin's lymphoma. It is clear that the latter group merges with leukaemia and the study of lymphoma-leukaemia has been hindered by the division of activities into departments of cytology, haematology and histopathology. The incidence of lymphoma is shown in Table 2, which records fewer cases of Hodgkin's disease than non-Hodgkin's lymphoma (NHL). Histiocytosis X has also been included in this group of diseases. It is considered that this is justified particularly as the immune system has been shown to play an increasing part in reticulo-endothelial neoplasia. Tumours in the "other reticulo-endothelial" group are rare and include chloroma and histiocytoses not fitting into the spectrum of histiocytosis X.
The presenting sites in 132 cases of NHL and Hodgkin's disease in the Manchester Children's Tumour Registry (MCTR) are compared in Table 3.
The distribution of NHL has some significance in relation to cell type. The T-cell tumours are more likely to have a mediastinal or thymic origin. The B-cell neoplasms arise more commonly below the diaphragm and are likely to involve the gastrointestinal tract although

* I am indebted to Mrs. B. Bartle for assistance with the preparation of the manuscript, to Mr. P. Fletcher for help with photomicrography and to Dr. J. M. Birch for help with the tables
1 The Manchester Children's Tumour Registry is supported by Cancer Research Campaign

Table 1. Frequency of leukaemias in the MCTR, 1954–1980

	Males	Females	Total	% group	% total tumours
Acute lymphoid leukaemia	411	289	700	79	26
Acute myeloid leukaemia	62	71	133	15	5
Acute monocytic leukaemia	6	14	20	2	1
Chronic myeloid leukaemia	9	5	14	2	1
Other	10	10	20	2	1
Total			887		33

Table 2. Frequency of lymphomas and other reticulo-endothelial tumours in the MCTR, 1954–1980

	Males	Females	Total	% group	% total tumours
Non-Hodgkin's lymphoma	83	42	125	41	5
Hodgkin's disease	71	30	101	33	4
Histiocytosis X	37	30	67	22	2
Other reticulo-endothelial	9	5	14	5	1
Total			307		11

Table 3. Presenting sites of NHL and Hodgkin's disease in the MCTR

Site	No. of cases	
	NHL	Hodgkin's disease
Cervical nodes	29	66
Cervical nodes and mediastinum	–	16
Mediastinum	23	5
Disseminated	24	12
Gastrointestinal tract	15	–
Abdominal nodes	14	–
Other nodes	10	–
Bone	7	–
Pharynx	5	–
Other	5	6
Total	132	105

pharyngeal lymphomas may be of either T-cell or B-cell origin. T-cell markers include acid phosphatase and receptors for sheep erythrocytes together with reaction with monoclonal antibodies. B-cell origin may be indicated by the demonstration of surface immunoglobulins. The B-cell lymphomas have been divided into Burkitt and non-Burkitt types based on clinical and cytological features, the latter including the uniformity of the tumour cells.

In the MCTR only one case has been regarded as justifying the diagnosis of Burkitt's lymphoma; it occurred in a fair-haired Caucasian boy with a lesion in the mandible giving rise to dislocation of the teeth. Non-Hodgkin's lymphoma presenting as a bone-destroying tumour is a feature of T-cell rather than B-cell disease, as reported by Dura et al. (1981). In this series one patient had a destructive lesion in the region of the knee-joint which was thought to be an osteosarcoma, and amputation was considered before biopsy was performed. The cases with disseminated or generalised distribution include T-cell and B-cell tumours although the latter would predominate in patients presenting with enlarged cervical lymph nodes.

Among the sites listed as "other" in Table 2 are two extradural tumours; similar neoplasms of B-cell origin are recorded by Dura et al. (1981).

The great majority of non-Hodgkin's lymphomas were histologically of diffuse type and this has been the experience generally reported. Lymphomas of nodular type do, however, occasionally occur in childhood; assessment of the material in the MCTR shows the incidence to be in the region of 2%.

The relationship between lymphoma and leukaemia has already been stressed; leukaemic conversion is more likely with T-cell tumours than with B-cell tumours.

A small number of immunoblastic lymphomas have been recorded in the MCTR. One tumour of B-cell origin was diagnosed in a boy with purine nucleoside phosphorylase deficiency (Watson et al. 1981). This association would support the suggestion of Lukes and Collins (1975) and Lennert et al. (1975) that there may be a relationship between immunological abnormalities and the development of immunoblastic lymphomas of B-cell type.

Hodgkin's disease showed a different clinical presentation, the majority of cases having involvement of the cervical nodes and/or mediastinum (Table 3).

Histologically, the cases of Hodgkin's disease showed mainly a lymphocyte-predominant and mixed cellularity pattern. Few examples of lymphocyte-depleted tumours were seen. Mediastinal involvement showed an equal sex incidence and was associated with a relatively high incidence of tumours with the histological nodular sclerosing features of disease.

Neuroblastoma

Neuroblastoma was the most frequently encountered solid tumour in the MCTR with 168 recorded cases (Table 4). The total number of cases of astrocytoma was rather higher but it does not seem to be justified to group the different types of this neoplasm together. It is probable that the incidence of neuroblastoma may be rather higher than recorded, as 11 of the tumours were found by chance at autopsy (Birch et al. 1980). All were grossly recognisable tumours, and did not include any classified as "neuroblastoma-in-situ". One of the patients was a microcephalic boy and this association is referred to by Miller et al. (1968) in their study of the epidemiology of neuroblastoma.

Male predominance was a feature in the MCTR cases (97 males and 71 females).

The neuroblastoma may show varying degrees of maturation towards its benign counterpart, the ganglioneuroma. However, all tumours with incomplete differentiation have been classified in this review as neuroblastomas to avoid cumbersome terminology. The benign ganglioneuroma was relatively rare, accounting for 8.6% of the group.

The distribution of benign and malignant tumours showed a rather different pattern (see Table 5).

Table 4. Frequency of other embryonal tumours in the MCTR, 1954–1980

	Males	Females	Total	% total tumours
Wilms' tumour	69	70	139	5
Neuroblastoma	97	71	168	6
Bilateral retinoblastoma	14	15	29 }	3
Unilateral retinoblastoma	24	25	49 }	
Hepatoblastoma	11	2	13	< 1

Table 5. Presenting sites of benign and malignant tumours in the MCTR

Site	No. of cases	
	Ganglioneuroma	Neuroblastoma
Adrenal	1	30
Abdominal retroperitoneal	4	61
Thorax	7	14
Cervical region	1	4
Pelvis	1	4
Spinal and dumb-bell	1	8
Leg	1	–
Total	16	121

There is a higher proportion of thoracic tumours in the benign group whereas the great majority of neuroblastomas were in the adrenal or retroperitoneal regions. Occasional examples of intracranial neuroblastoma have been recorded (Ojeda et al. 1980) but no such case has been included in the MCTR.

The neuroblastoma is a tumour of infancy and early childhood and has a particular tendency to spread to bone marrow, lymph nodes and liver. The sites of metastases differ with age, with older patients having bone without liver involvement and the reverse pattern being seen in infancy (Marsden 1963). Diffuse infiltration is a particular feature in young infants and the concept of IV-S neuroblastoma has been proposed by Evans et al. (1980) with the possibility of multiple primary sites rather than metastatic spread. In the series of Evans et al. nearly half of the patients with liver involvement showed resolution of lesions without treatment. Skin deposits are another feature of infants with neuroblastoma and this is also true of the young patient with leukaemia.

The histological differentiation towards the neurone must be taken into account in prognosis (Hughes et al. 1974). A large number of neurosecretory granules seen on electron microscopy may be associated with a more favourable excretion pattern (Romansky et al. 1978). The presence of rosettes does not, however, have any favourable implication. Serum immunoglobulin levels may also be related to survival (Sawada et al. 1979); these authors found elevation of IgG but not of IgA or IgM to be significant. Phaeochromocytoma is a rare tumour in childhood and only three examples have been recorded in the MCTR. During the period under review there were also four tumours of the carotid and aortic bodies.

Table 6. Frequency of intracranial tumours in the MCTR, 1954–1980

	Males	Females	Total	% group	% total tumours
Juvenile astrocytoma	71	76	147	24	5
Other astrocytoma	50	45	95	15	4
Ependymoma	33	40	73	12	3
Medulloblastoma	86	48	134	22	5
Other glioma	17	10	27	4	1
Craniopharyngioma	14	13	27	4	1
Meningioma	4	8	12	2	< 1
Other intracranial	7	11	18	3	1
Unbiopsied	44	42	86	14	3
Total			619		23

Tumours of the Central Nervous System

The central nervous system is the most common presenting site (22.3%) of childhood tumours (Birch et al. 1980).

Juvenile astrocytoma (5%) and medulloblastoma (5%) are the most numerically important solid neoplasms after neuroblastoma, and together with adult astrocytoma and ependymoma account for the majority of intracranial tumours (Table 6).

The juvenile astrocytoma should be separated from the "other" or adult tumours not only on histological grounds but also by their site of origin and clinical behaviour (Table 7). The juvenile neoplasms predominate in the cerebellum and in the region of the hypothalamus; they are relatively uncommon in the cerebral hemispheres and brain-stem where the adult tumours tend to be found. Both types of astrocytoma are seen in the cerebellum but 77% of the lesions at this site were juvenile.

Patients with juvenile tumours may survive for many years without further treatment as long as the circulation of the cerebrospinal fluid is maintained. It is important to classify astrocytomas histologically before trying to assess the results of therapy. The adult tumours show a broad spectrum of malignancy, from relatively low grade neoplasms to highly aggressive glioblastomas.

The great majority of medulloblastomas are cerebellar and involve the vermis. They seed throughout the ventricular system following blockage of the fourth ventricle and may show extensive spread into the spinal theca. In addition, more than 80 examples of extracranial metastases have been recorded (Pollak et al. 1981). These authors report a patient with extensive skeletal involvement who was treated as a case of leukaemia for one year.

The histological features of the medulloblastoma have led to attempts to subdivide this group of tumours. There is one case of definite medullomyoblastoma in the MCTR, with clearly defined striated fibres, and this diagnosis has been previously considered on a few occasions. However, from the very limited experience gained it would seem that the medullomyoblastoma does not behave differently from the medulloblastoma and that spinal thecal involvement occurs (Fig. 1).

Twelve per cent of intracranial tumours in the MCTR were ependymomas and together with astrocytoma and medulloblastoma accounted for nearly threequarters of the neoplasms of the central nervous system. It is possible that this figure would have been

Table 7. Sites of origin of astrocytomas in the MCTR

Site	No. of cases	
	Juvenile astrocytoma	Adult astrocytoma
Cerebrum	12	43
Cerebellum	55	16
Brain-stem	8	26
Spinal cord	5	3
Third ventricle	22	–
Mixed site	2	–
Total	94	88

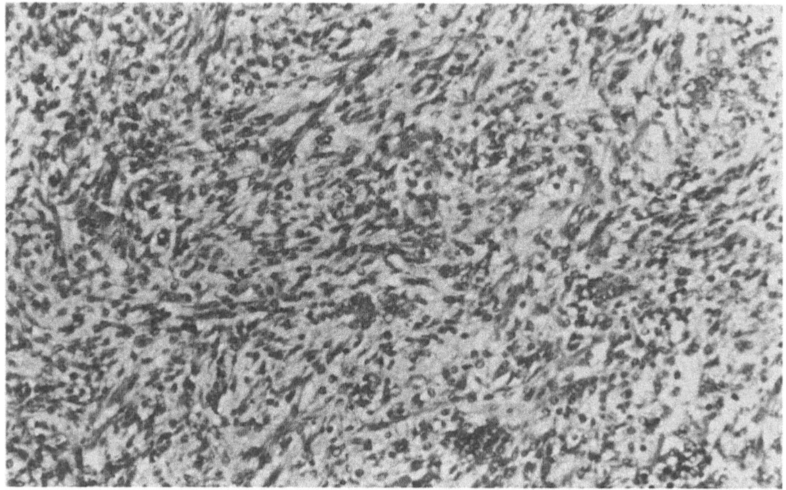

Fig. 1. Medullomyoblastoma showing small cells with striated muscle fibres. H&E. Objective × 10

even higher when it is considered that 86 (14%) of the lesions were not biopsied. The reasons for including such cases have been discussed elsewhere (Marsden and Steward 1976) and to exclude such patients would give an incomplete picture of the incidence of central nervous system tumours.

The great majority of ependymomas were in the region of the fourth ventricle often arising in the lateral angles, invading the cerebellum and extending down alongside the brain-stem and upper spinal cord. Of 74 consecutive tumours, 51 were infratentorial, with 20 in the cerebrum. The latter were noted in the parietal and frontal regions in particular but were sometimes widespread and accounted for the largest cerebral neoplasms in infants and younger patients. There were three spinal ependymomas with one myxopapillary tumour of the cauda equina.

Extracranial metastases, although not recorded in the MCTR, do occasionally occur with ependymomas and the author has seen a patient with pulmonary deposits following such a tumour.

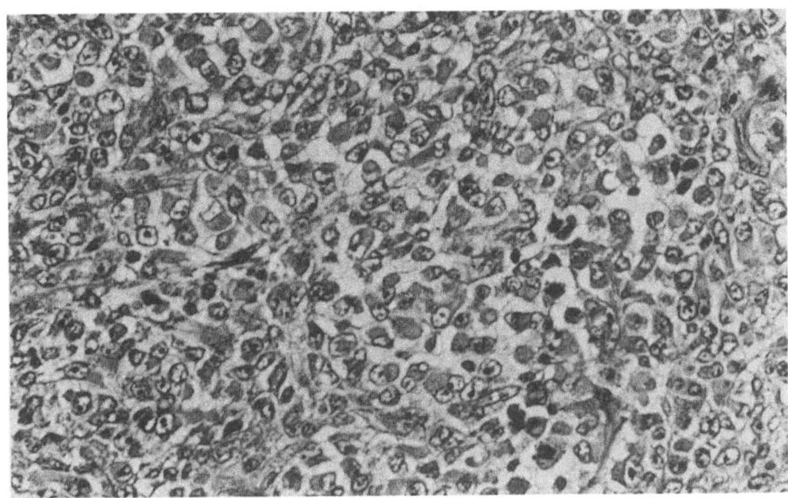

Fig. 2. "Rhabdoid" renal tumour with cells having abundant eosinophilic cytoplasm. H&E. Objective × 20

Renal Tumours

The Wilms' tumour is by far the commonest renal neoplasm in childhood and accounted for 5% of the total cases in the MCTR. Renal carcinomas, three of the clear cell type and one papillary, make up a small proportion of neoplasms, with mesoblastic nephroma and the bone-metastasising tumour showing a roughly similar incidence. Polygonal celled tumours, sometimes with a "rhabdoid" appearance and showing cytoplasmic fibrillary features on ultrastructural study (Haas et al. 1981) have been rare in the MCTR material (Figs. 2, 3, 4).

The histological range of the Wilms' tumour is broad but has a definite pattern. At one end of the range there is undifferentiated blastema often in a jigsaw pattern and separated by loose mesenchyme, though varying degrees of metanephric differentiation may be seen with regimentation of cells and tubular and glomerular structures. Mesodermal features may be prominent, particularly striated muscle, and at the other end of the range cartilage, bone, fat and squamous and columnar secretory epithelium may be noted, sometimes with cyst formation. The tumours differ from teratomata in that the tissues are differentiated, organoid development is not seen and the prominent central nervous tissue of the teratoma is not noted.

The presence of dysplastic lesions, which may regress and sclerose, was noted in about 20% of the kidneys which contained Wilms' tumours in the MCTR series. This feature was more commonly seen in bilateral than in unilateral tumours. The incidence of bilateral tumours was just over 4% with six examples in the 139 cases.

The prognosis in the Wilms' tumour is related to tubular differentiation (Lawler et al. 1975) which has some relation to, but is independent from, staging. The presence of other features such as glomeruli is less relevant.

With the greatly improved prognosis in the past few decades the search has been transferred from good prognostic histological features to the identification of adverse ones which may be present in the relatively few cases which do not respond to treatment. In this context the presence of pleomorphism or anaplasia (Beckwith and Palmer 1978) is an

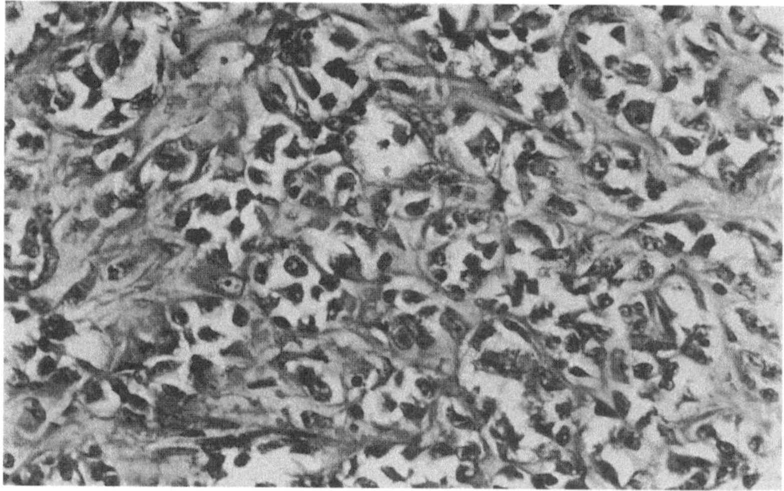

Fig. 3. "Rhabdoid" renal tumour with typical sclerotic pattern. H&E. Objective × 20

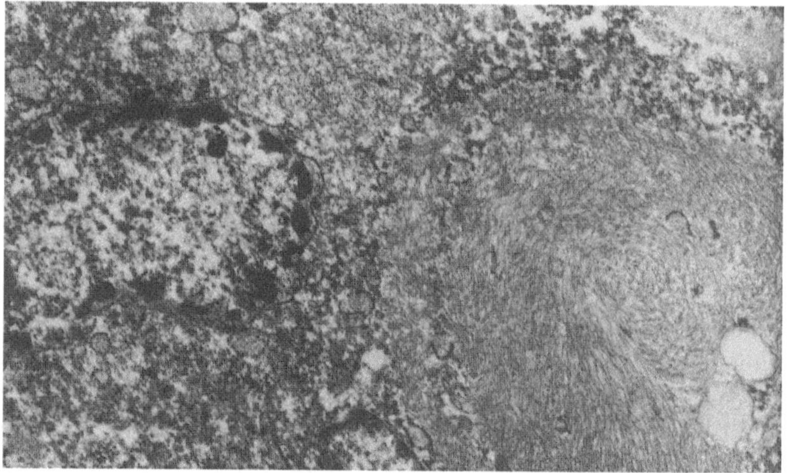

Fig. 4. Electronmicrograph of "rhabdoid" tumour showing fibrillary cytoplasmic inclusion. Uranylacetate lead citrate. Objective × 8,000

adverse indicator which overrides the favourable evidence of tubular differentiation (Fig. 5).

The bone-metastasising renal tumour pattern is a bad prognostic feature (Marsden and Lawler 1980) and is associated with the development of osseous deposits in about two-thirds of cases (Fig. 6). The high male predominance associated with this tumour is also different from that seen in the usual Wilms' tumours which, in the MCTR, occurred in 69 males and 70 females. In the bad prognostic group of renal tumours the polygonal cell or "rhabdoid" pattern has also been included. This neoplasm is less clearly defined as being of purely renal origin and similar histological features have been recorded in two MCTR

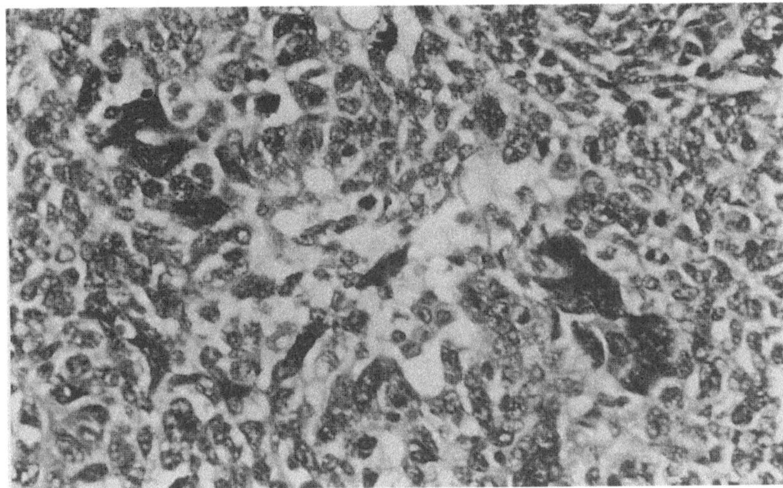

Fig. 5. Wilms' tumour showing pleomorphism with cells having bizarre nuclei. H&E. Objective × 20

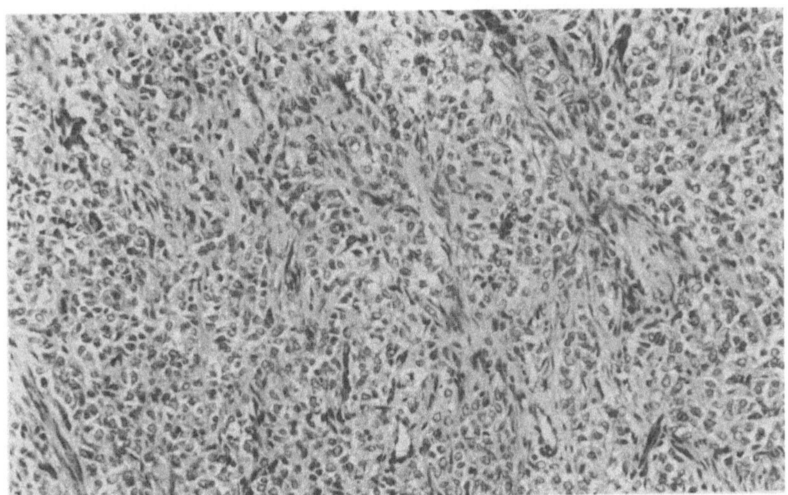

Fig. 6. Bone-metastasising renal tumour of childhood with polygonal cells, capillaries and interspersed fibrillary areas. H&E. Objective × 10

neoplasms of the head and neck region. These extrarenal "rhabdoid" tumours were clinically aggressive and resistant to chemotherapy.

Lymphoma, leiomyosarcoma and neuroblastoma may also present as renal neoplasms (Marsden et al. 1980).

The few cases of mesoblastic nephroma in the MCTR have all behaved in a benign manner and this has been the author's experience in general. However, Gonzalez-Crussi et al. (1981) in a study of eight cases of mesenchymal tumour of the infant kidney describe typical, malignant and intermediate cellular mesoblastic nephromas and report lung metastases in the two malignant cases in their series.

Table 8. Frequency of connective tissue tumours in the MCTR, 1954–1980

	Males	Females	Total	% group	% total tumours
Rhabdomyosarcoma	60	40	100	36	4
Fibrosarcoma	11	8	19	7	1
Synovial sarcoma	8	1	9	3	< 1
Osteosarcoma	30	38	68	24	3
Ewing's tumour	26	28	54	19	2
Other connective tissue tumours	15	13	28	10	1
Total			278		10

Bone and Soft Tissue Tumours

The rhabdomyosarcoma (RMS), osteosarcoma and Ewing's tumour account for 79% of the tumours in this group with the RMS being numerically the most important as shown in Table 8.

There are a number of other neoplasms in the connective tissue group but these are relatively rare and it is difficult to obtain sufficient material for study without collaboration between different centres.

The RMS in childhood is, for the most part, an embryonal mesenchymal tumour in which myoblastic differentiation may occur. Such differentiation is not to be expected in all neoplasms and this applies to 15% of tumours in the MCTR material. The myoblastic and non-myoblastic tumours are, however, identical in other respects and the term RMS has been used to include neoplasms which might otherwise be classified as embryonal sarcoma. In addition, electron microscopy and peroxidase staining for the detection of myoglobin has not been used in all cases and so the incidence of myoblastic differentiation could have been higher than has been recorded.

Adult or pleomorphic tumours arising from muscle are rare in childhood and account for 3% of the group in the MCTR.

Histologically, the embryonal tumours may appear loose or dense and may show botryoid features; other neoplasms are classified as alveolar RMS. In a recent analysis alveolar tumours accounted for 17% of the group and were found in rather older children than were the other types of embryonal RMS (Fig. 7). The head and neck and pelvic regions were the main sites for RMS with relatively fewer tumours in the peripheral muscles, abdomen, testis and bile duct. Spread to lymph nodes has been recorded in about one third of cases in the MCTR with lung metastases in 20% and deposits less commonly seen in brain, liver and bone. There may be widespread disease and extensive involvement of the skeleton may occur. Involvement of the central nervous system is a particular hazard with neoplasms in the aural and pharyngeal regions.

The other soft tissue tumours are relatively rare in childhood. Only 19 cases of fibrosarcoma have been recorded in the same period as 100 cases of RMS. Four of the fibrosarcomas were congenital or infantile and may belong to a distinct group. Gonzalez-Crussi et al. (1980) describe primitive cells with a myxoid stroma and suggest the presence of a histiocytic component in these congenital tumours. Metastases are unusual in the fibrosarcoma and were noted in 16% of cases in the group, or 20% if the congenital tumours are excluded. The neoplasms are, however, locally invasive and two highly

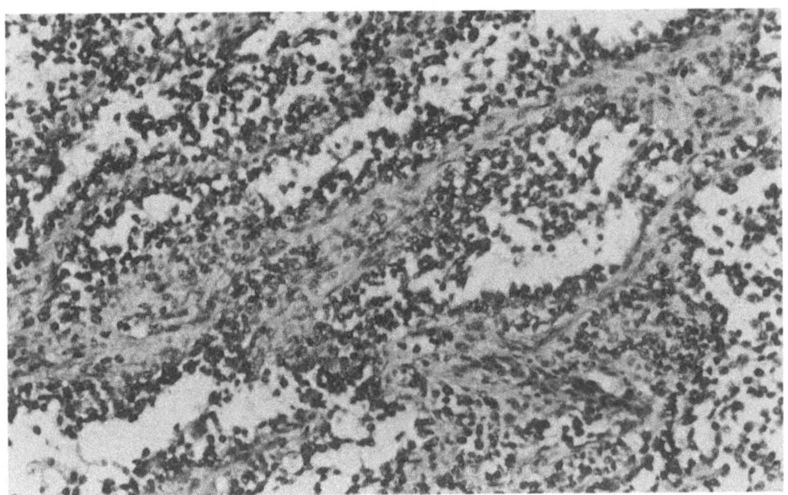

Fig. 7. Alveolar rhabdomyosarcoma with fibrous, septa and spaces lined by tumour cells. H&E. Objective × 10

aggressive fibrosarcomas of the face have been recorded, being particularly difficult to treat and possibly belonging to a distinct tumour entity.

Apart from synovial sarcoma (nine cases) and haemangiopericytoma (seven cases) the material in the MCTR is insufficient to make possible any assessment of the behaviour of the remaining neoplasms in the soft tissue group. Small numbers of fibrous histiocytoma, alveolar soft part sarcoma, liposarcoma, angiosarcoma and mesenchymoma have been included. The term mesenchymoma has been used according to Stout's definition (1948), being applied to a tumour which contains two or more mesodermal tissues excluding fibrous tissue. The tumour appears to be more frequently diagnosed in the United States than in Manchester (Marsden 1982). The rare liposarcomas in childhood are highly differentiated and cause problems by virtue of their size and situation rather than by any tendency to metastasise.

The synovial sarcomas in the MCTR have all been biphasic tumours, although Mickelson et al. (1980) consider monophasic synovial tumours to have particular ultrastructural features. Lymph node metastases constituted the most common method of spread in the tumours reviewed in Manchester, followed by lung, bone and liver deposits.

The haemangiopericytomas had a double peak age incidence, being seen in infants or preadolescent children. The tumour is more common in adults, with paediatric cases accounting for only about 10% of total incidence.

The behaviour of the haemangiopericytomas in the MCTR was difficult to predict from their histological appearances. The tendency to recur after excision was a prominent feature but the incidence of metastases was relatively low.

The tumours of bone were mainly osteosarcoma and Ewing's tumour with slight preponderance of the former. In the 68 osteosarcomas shown in Table 8 the majority (50% or 74%) occurred in long bones of the leg. There were 12 tumours in the long bones of the arm (18%) and a few tumours arose in the thoracic cage and pelvis. One osteosarcoma developed in the frontal region of the skull following treatment for retinoblastoma, emphasising the association between these neoplasms. Another osteosarcoma was found in the frontal lobe of the brain with no apparent connection with the skull and no evidence to suggest that it was a metastatic tumour.

The Ewing's tumour did not show the same preponderance for the long bones of the leg although this was the commonest primary site, with 19 of 54 cases (37%). Fifteen tumours of the upper limb accounted for 27% of cases and 11 tumours (21%) were recorded in the pelvic bones. There were six neoplasms in the thoracic cage with occasional examples in the bones of the vertebral column and foot. No case of primary Ewing's tumour was recorded in the bones of the skull although this was not an unusual site for metastases. The differential diagnosis between Ewing's tumour and metastatic neuroblastoma has been discussed by Marsden and Steward (1964), who described a greater tendency for infiltration of the surrounding soft tissues in the former. Ewing's tumour has been classified into typical and atypical types on an ultrastructural basis using variability in cell size and the presence or absence of cytoplasmic organelles (Llombart-Bosch et al. 1978).

Germ Cell and Other Rare Tumours

The tumours of germ cell origin comprise a relatively small but important group of childhood tumours. The cases listed in Table 9 include only those considered to be malignant. They differ from other paediatric neoplasms in that their incidence is greater in females. The ovary is the most common site of origin and sacro-coccygeal teratomas are also more common in the female. The sacro-coccygeal region is the second most frequent site of germ cell tumours in childhood, followed by the testis and the intracranial region. Small numbers are seen at a variety of other sites from the neck to the pelvis, usually, but not invariably, in the midline. Occasional neoplasms have been recorded in the spinal canal.

Germ cell tumours were classified in the MCTR into benign and malignant teratoma, germinoma, yolk-sac tumour, choriocarcinoma and mixed neoplasms. In a small number of cases it was difficult to be certain on histological grounds whether the tumours were benign or malignant. In this context, the presence of undifferentiated elements appeared to be more significant in older children than in infants. In a study of 137 germ cell tumours of childhood in the MCTR (Marsden et al. 1981) yolk-sac elements were present in all the sacro-coccygeal, testicular and abdominal tumours which proved fatal (Fig. 8). Other neoplasms caused problems because of their situation, as with tumours involving the heart or central nervous system. Malignant behaviour was, however, encountered in ovarian tumours which did not have a yolk-sac component. Germinomas were confined to the ovary and intracranial regions, benign teratomas were mainly ovarian and sacro-coccygeal but the yolk-sac tumour had its highest incidence in the testis.

This section includes other relatively uncommon and rare paediatric neoplasms. In the former category would be placed the hepatoblastoma, with 13 cases in the MCTR, and nasopharyngeal carcinoma (12 cases). Hepatoblastoma is of interest because of the association with growth disorders and other tumours. Nasopharyngeal carcinoma is of special importance because of its geographical distribution and its association with the Epstein-Barr virus. Adrenal tumours were difficult to assess in respect of their expected behaviour based on their histological features. There were 12 examples, three being regarded as benign and nine showing malignant features to a varying degree. All the patients with tumours classified as benign are alive without recurrence but five of the nine other patients have died.

Table 9. Frequency of germ cell and other rare tumours in the MCTR, 1954–1980

	Males	Females	Total	% total tumours
Teratoma and yolk-sac tumour	18	32	50	2
Germinoma	6	11	17	1
Epithelial tumours	32	27	59	2
Unbiopsied extracranial tumours	9	11	20	1
Other rare tumours	6	9	15	1
Unclassified tumours	22	16	38	1

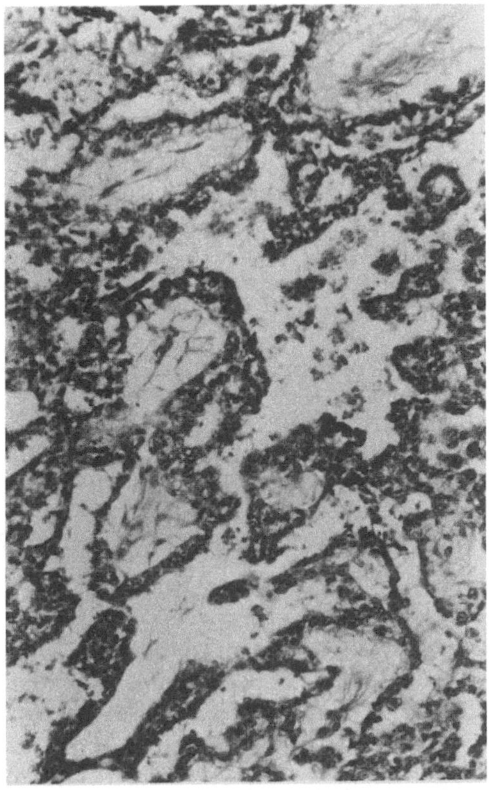

Fig. 8. Yolk-sac tumour with Schiller-Duval bodies having central capillaries and a coronet of tumour cells. H&E. Objective × 10

Carcinomas are rare in childhood, and only a few have been recorded in the MCTR — thyroid 3, bronchus 3, large bowel 3, salivary gland 2, ileum 1, ovary 1. Only one example of carcinoma of the breast has been seen, an intraduct, non-infiltrating lesion with favourable outcome. During the same period there were nine examples of fibroadenoma of the breast, none of which occurred before puberty.

Naevi and malignant melanoma may also cause problems in diagnosis.

Although malignant melanoma is rare in childhood, seven cases were recorded in the MCTR, three of which were in the head and neck region.

Isolated examples of other rare tumours have been noted in the present series but their low incidence made it impossible to assess their natural history. Inter-centre cooperation is required to classify these very rare tumours and to define their behaviour.

The relatively small number of cases of childhood cancer allow the investigator to make detailed observations on many aspects including genetic, geographical, epidemiological and immunological features related to both larger and smaller groups of neoplasms. More complete identification of particular tumour entities is also needed. In conclusion, considering the relatively small part external carcinogens apparently play in the aetiology of childhood cancer, the subject is particularly suitable for studying the more subtle relationships which may be implicated in carcinogenesis.

References

1. Beckwith JB, Palmer NF (1978) Histology and prognosis of Wilms' tumour. Results from the first national Wilms' tumour study. Cancer 41: 1937–1948
2. Birch JM, Marsden HB, Swindell R (1980) Incidence of malignant disease in childhood: a 24-year review of the Manchester Children's Tumour Registry data. Br J Cancer 42: 215–223
3. Dura WT, Gladkowska-Dura MJ, Johnson WW (1981) Non-Hodgkin's lymphoma in the first two decades. Morphologic and immunocytochemical study. Virchows Archiv [Pathol Anat] 390: 23–62
4. Evans AE, D'Angio GJ, Gerson JM, Robinson J, Schnaufer L (1980) A review of IV-S neuroblastoma patients at the Children's Hospital of Philadelphia. Cancer 45: 833–839
5. Gonzalez-Crussi F, Wiederhold MD, Sotelo-Avila C (1980) Congenital fibrosarcoma. Presence of a histiocytic component. Cancer 46: 77–86
6. Gonzalez-Crussi F, Sotelo-Avila C, Kidd JM (1981) Mesenchymal renal tumours in infancy: a reappraisal. Hum Pathol 12: 78–85
7. Haas JE, Palmer NF, Weinberg AG, Beckwith JB (1981) Ultrastructure of malignant rhabdoid tumour of kidney. Hum Pathol 12: 646–657
8. Hughes M, Marsden HB, Palmer MK (1974) Neuroblastoma – relation of histology to prognosis and clinical staging. Cancer 34: 1706–1711
9. Lawler W, Marsden HB, Palmer MR (1975) Wilms' tumour – histologic variation and prognosis. Cancer 36: 1122–1126
10. Lennert K, Stein H, Kaiserling E (1975) Cytological and functional criteria for the classification of malignant lymphomata. Br J Cancer 31 (Suppl II): 29–35
11. Llombart-Bosch A, Blache R, Peydro-Olaya A (1978) Ultrastructural study of 28 cases of Ewing's sarcoma: typical and atypical forms. Cancer 41: 1362–1373
12. Lukes RJ, Collins RD (1975) New approach to the classification of lymphomata. Br J Cancer (Suppl II) 31: 1–28
13. Marsden HB (1963) Clinical and pathological features of neuroblastoma. In: Varley H, Gowenlock AH (eds) The clinical chemistry of monoamines. Elsevier Publishing Company, Amsterdam London New York
14. Marsden HB The pathology of soft tissue sarcomas. In: D'Angio G, Evans AE (eds) Bone and soft tissue sarcomas. Edward Arnold, London (in press)
15. Marsden HB, Steward JK (1964) Ewing's tumour and neuroblastoma. J Clin Pathol 17: 411–417
16. Marsden HB, Steward JK (eds) (1976) Tumours in children. Springer, Berlin Heidelberg New York
17. Marsden HB, Lennox EL, Lawler W, Kinnier-Wilson LM (1980) Bone metastases in childhood renal tumours. Br J Cancer 41: 875–879
18. Marsden HB, Lawler W (1980) Bone-metastasizing renal tumour of childhood. Histopathological and clinical review of 38 cases. Virchows Archiv [Pathol Anat] 387: 341–351

19. Marsden HB, Birch JM, Swindell R (1981) Germ cell tumours of childhood: a review of 137 cases. J Clin Pathol 34: 879–883
20. Mickelson MR, Brown SA, Maynard JA, Cooper RR, Bonfiglio M (1980) Synovial sarcoma. An EM study of monophasic and biphasic forms. Cancer 45: 2109–2118
21. Miller RW, Fraumeni JF Jr, Hill JA (1968) Neuroblastoma: epidemiologic approach to its origin. Am J Dis Child 115: 253–261
22. Ojeda VJ, Jacobsen PF, Papadimitriou JM (1980) Primary cerebral neuroblastoma. Case report with light microscopy, tissue culture and EM study. Pathology 12: 269–274
23. Pollak ER, Miller JH, Vye MV (1981) Medulloblastoma presenting as leukaemia. Am J Clin Pathol 76: 98–103
24. Romansky SG, Crocker DW, Shaw KNF (1978) Ultrastructural studies on neuroblastoma. Cancer 42: 2392–2398
25. Sawada T, Suginoto TS, Tazawa M, Takada H, Kusunoki T (1979) Serum immunoglobulin levels in patients with neuroblastoma and their prognosis. J Pediat Surg 14: 405–413
26. Stout AP (1948) Myxoma. The tumor of primitive mesenchyme. Mesenchymoma, the mixed tumor of mesenchymal derivatives. Ann Surg 127: 278–290
27. Watson AR, Evans DIK, Marsden HB, Miller V, Rogers PA (1981) Purine nucleoside phosphorylase deficiency associated with a fatal lymphoproliferative disorder. Arch Dis Child 56: 563–565

Assessment by Radiological Techniques

E. M. Sweet

Royal Hospital for Sick Children, Glasgow G3 8SJ, United Kingdom

Introduction — Available Techniques

Rapidly changing technology has increased the diagnostic radiologist's involvement in paediatric oncology as "radiology" has expanded to include ultrasound and nuclear medicine.

Organ imaging techniques are divided, from the patient's point of view, into two categories — invasive and non-invasive. When dealing with malignant disease this is a more realistic division than separating those using ionising radiations from those which do not. A recent paper (Faulkner and Moores 1982) reported high doses of scattered radiation near CT scanners, indicating a possible hazard to nurses acting regularly as parent-substitutes to children undergoing computed tomography. This fact must be considered when implementing the policy of having a parent or familiar parent-substitute with the child throughout diagnostic procedures, which are inevitably frightening experiences.

Non-invasive x-ray examinations comprise conventional radiography, conventional tomography and computed tomography of the lungs. Invasive x-ray examinations involve injections of iodine-containing contrast media for intravenous urography, myelography, arteriography or enhanced computed tomography, or introduction of barium into the alimentary tract, usually with air to produce double contrast for mucosal detail.

The confidence of the pioneers in the use of ultrasound in its safety has been confirmed; at diagnostic frequencies it is free from biological risk to patients, operators or assistants. The main disadvantages are that ultrasound is reflected by air in lungs and by intestinal gas, which is hard to clear from the paediatric abdomen. It is also more demanding on radiologists' time than many other investigations.

Isotopes, with few exceptions, are injected intravenously but produce relatively low radiation doses.

While the prospect of nuclear magnetic resonance as a non-invasive technique is exciting there are as yet no reports of its use in paediatric oncology and the formidable appearance of the apparatus in its present form suggests that problems may be encountered in persuading children to enter without heavy sedation or general anaesthesia.

Choice of Technique for Organ Imaging

Organ imaging in paediatric oncology has four purposes:

1. Establishing diagnosis;
2. Staging known disease;

Recent Results in Cancer Research. Vol. 88
© Springer-Verlag Berlin · Heidelberg 1983

3. Monitoring treatment, including complications;
4. Following up after completion of treatment.

In choosing the appropriate facility simple investigations should be done first and the more expensive, more invasive and less readily available should be used where indicated rather than routinely.

Establishing the Diagnosis

Definitive diagnosis in oncology involves histology, but diagnostic imaging can suggest the diagnosis and indicate the most likely source of tissue for its confirmation, often after relatively few investigations. A child presenting with pallor and lethargy may on penetrated chest x-ray and an anteroposterior x-ray of the knees show changes almost certainly associated with leukaemia. They include mediastinal enlargement in T-cell leukaemia and broad radiolucent bands across distal femoral and proximal tibial metaphyses in "common" acute lymphoblastic leukaemia (Sweet and Willoughby 1980) (Fig. 1). Similarly, an intravenous urogram on a child with an abdominal mass may present features almost pathognomonic of neuroblastoma (Fig. 2) or Wilms' tumour or nephroblastoma (Fig. 3) sufficient for diagnosis. With the increasing popularity of percutaneous biopsy techniques for tissue diagnosis, x-ray fluoroscopy with image intensification, ultrasound and even computed tomography are being used to locate appropriate biopsy sites during the procedure. Arteriography is rarely necessary for diagnosis and may now be reserved for therapeutic embolisation which has been used occasionally to reduce massive Wilms' tumours to operable dimensions (Danis et al. 1979).

Staging

The current rapid progress in the more rational selection of treatment of children with cancer requires detailed pretreatment assessment and accurate staging of the disease before specific treatment is decided upon. The demands made on diagnostic imaging services in the current United Kingdom therapeutic trials in childhood malignancy are moderate. Simple radiological examinations are mandatory and those not generally available are optional in most cases. Accessibility of specialised equipment and local expertise in its use are important in planning staging procedures.
Inevitably as each new diagnostic technique is developed its application to malignant disease is investigated with enthusiasm. Eventually this enthusiasm becomes tempered in the light of experience and only then can the temptation to request or even demand every available mode in every patient be rationally resisted. Local circumstances will dictate local practice and although major cancer centres will have access to all modes of investigation expertise will vary and not all modes may be available in a single hospital.
Paediatric hospital departments have a unique atmosphere to which children respond, unlike that of larger diagnostic imaging departments in general hospitals, where children are only occasional visitors. This produces problems in patient cooperation not necessarily overcome by sending along parents or nursing and medical staff with whom the child is familiar. Results may be degraded and general anaesthesia may even be required where with less profound sedation satisfactory results would confidently be anticipated in paediatric hospital departments. The current recommendations for investigating metastatic disease are summarised in Table 1.

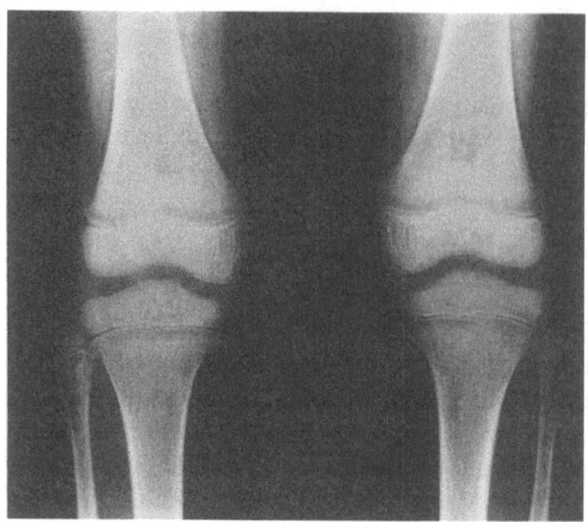

Fig. 1. "Common" acute lymphoblastic leukaemia. Knees show broad radiolucent bands across femoral, tibial and fibular metaphyses

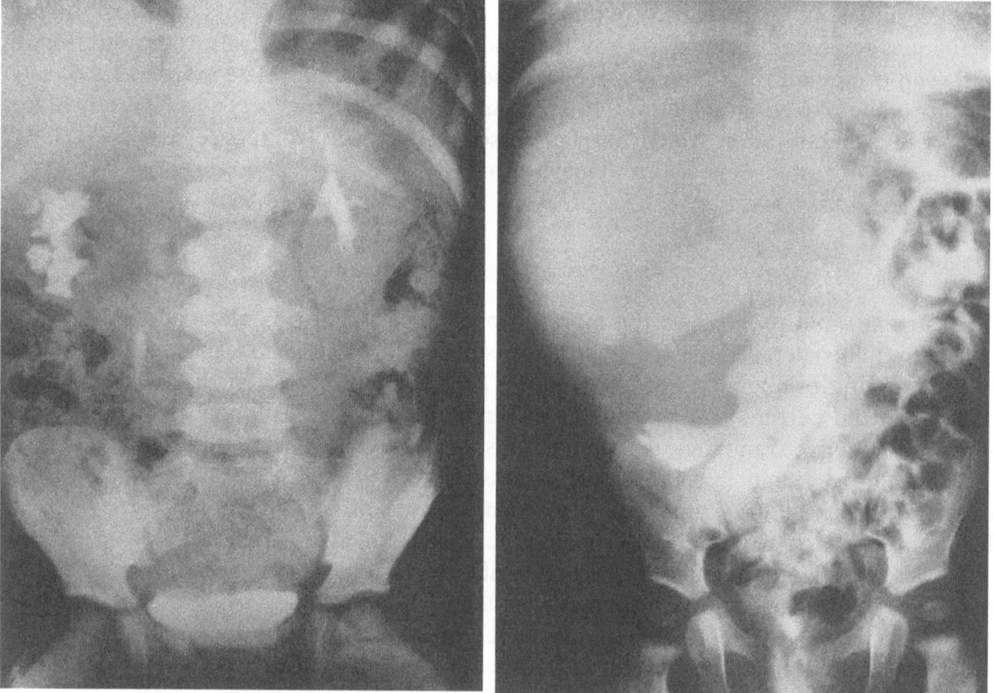

Fig. 2 (left). Neuroblastoma. Intravenous urogram with calcification superior and medial to right kidney which is slightly obstructed and displaced infero-laterally

Fig. 3 (right). Nephroblastoma. Dilated distorted pyelogram in enlarged right kidney which crosses midline. Left kidney removed earlier for nephroblastoma

Table 1. Most promising investigation related to site of suspected metastatic disease

Tumour site	Radiological investigation
Thorax	Computed tomography
Liver	Ultrasound, radioisotope or computed tomography
Lymph node structure below diaphragm	Bipedal lymphangiography
Lymph node enlargement	Computed tomography
Inferior vena cava	Ultrasound
Skeleton	Radioisotope
Intracranial, intraspinal	Computed tomography
Retroperitoneum	Computed tomography

Computed Tomography

There is no rival to computed tomography for the investigation of intracranial tumours. Equally accurate results have been obtained in investigating spinal tumours, both primary and metastatic, by combining computed tomography with metrizamide myelography (Resjo et al. 1979; Harwood-Nash 1981). The relative rigidity of the cranial vault makes examination of its contents and the surrounding tissues easier in children than examination of the chest and abdomen, where respiratory movements may cause problems unless the most up-to-date fast-speed scanners are available or general anaesthesia is employed. Computed tomography will illustrate diffuse organ enlargement or organ displacement by tumour masses and will isolate masses within organs provided they are of different tissue density and over a certain size, which in the case of the lungs is 3 mm. This suggests that computed tomography is more sensitive than whole lung tomography (Husband and Golding 1982). Reports disputing this sensitivity in comparison with conventional four-view chest radiography and whole lung tomography (Smoger et al. 1982) are attributable to use of less up-to-date computed tomography apparatus. However, due to the heavy clinical demands on whole body scanners, computed tomography of the lungs should be restricted to the investigation of those children whose lesions are likely to involve the lungs but in whom conventional radiography and whole lung tomography have failed to demonstrate any abnormality.

Retroperitoneal tumours are well illustrated by computed tomography (Kuhns 1981) and it may sometimes be the most rewarding investigation (Laurin et al. 1981).

Nuclear Medicine

Nuclear medicine is recommended as the most sensitive investigation for establishing skeletal involvement in malignant disease, most lesions being vascular and showing as "hot" spots of increased isotope uptake (Gilday et al. 1977). In assessing skeletal involvement, where facilities are readily available conventional x-ray examination of suspicious areas should follow a preliminary isotope survey, to exclude false positive results related to trauma or to other diseases. If isotope examination is less accessible it can be reserved for those children who, although showing so evidence of skeletal involvement on conventional radiography, have diseases such as neuroblastoma which may have

asymptomatic skeletal involvement (Howman-Giles et al. 1979). However, children with evidence of skeletal deposits as shown by isotope survey usually have changes demonstrable by x-ray, although the extent of involvement demonstrated may vary with the different techniques (Carty 1982).
Isotope examination is essential in the staging of primary bone tumours; soft tissue extensions and intramedullary spread are well illustrated and at surgery are found to correspond accurately to what has been determined by this technique. Similar accuracy has been claimed for computed tomography (Tschappeler and Vock 1982). Isotopes are also valuable in detecting bone metastases in patients with osteogenic sarcoma and in staging bone metastasising nephroblastomas (Appell et al. 1982).

Ultrasound Imaging

Being non-invasive and available in most diagnostic imaging departments ultrasound is particularly useful in assessing intra-abdominal masses involving the liver and kidneys (Jaffe et al. 1981). A sonar scan may be the only investigation required to confirm the findings of an intravenous urogram performed after conventional scout x-rays. It is particularly useful in differentiating liver enlargement from displacement and is as accurate in assessing liver pathology as nuclear medicine and computed tomography. As it shows both invasion and displacement it gives a more accurate demonstration of involvement of the inferior vena cava than do computed tomography and intravenous contrast cavography (Slovis et al. 1981).
Ultrasound is also accurate in assessing pelvic pathology (Fig. 4) but due to reflection by bowel gas shadows it is of limited value in staging retroperitoneal disease between the epigastrium and the true pelvis. Computed tomography is more reliable at these sites.

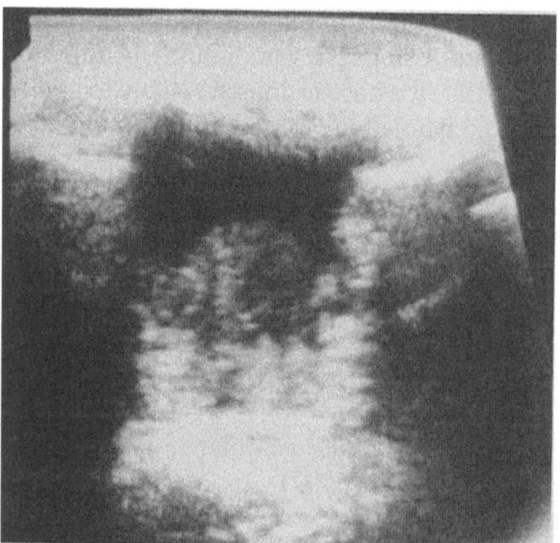

Fig. 4. Rhabdomyosarcoma of bladder. Transverse sonar scan showing echogenic tumour tissue in and posterior to posterior bladder wall encroaching anteriorly into cavity of well filled bladder with echofree urine

Lymphography

Bipedal lymphangiography with iodine-containing oily media is useful in demonstrating lesions in lymph nodes which may not necessarily be enlarged. Computed tomography on the other hand, will demonstrate lymph node enlargement and may show enlarged nodes not filled at lymphography, particularly in the upper abdomen. The examinations are therefore complementary rather than optional alternatives.

For the staging of intra-abdominal lymphomas and soft tissue sarcomas of lower limbs and pelvis both examinations are recommended. Unfortunately, lymph node contrast disappears rapidly in children, usually well within a year of lymphography, limiting its usefulness in assessing the long term response of diseased lymph nodes to treatment.

Monitoring Response to Treatment

In assessing the response to treatment of disease, it may be necessary to repeat the investigations which gave worthwhile information at the time of diagnosis. Again, those modes which are least invasive and most readily accessible should be considered first. For example, while simple penetrated chest x-rays will be sufficient to monitor mediastinal disease in most patients, the investigation of intracranial lesions will require computed tomography, as will follow-up of intra-abdominal lymph node enlargement (Blackledge et al. 1981). If ultrasonic volumetric measurements are satisfactory at the initial assessment of intra-abdominal neuroblastoma (Figs. 5, 6), the same technique should be used for follow-up. Computed tomography should be reserved for cases inadequately demonstrated by ultrasound examination. Chest x-rays are performed at intervals determined by the natural history of the primary tumour, to demonstrate possible metastatic deposits in the lungs. If negative, they should be supplemented by computed tomography of the thorax in cases where the demonstration of lung metastases would influence the policy of treatment. The recommended intervals are listed in Table 2. Some nodules appear which are not malignant deposits, but these are usually distinguishable with care (Cohen et al. 1982).

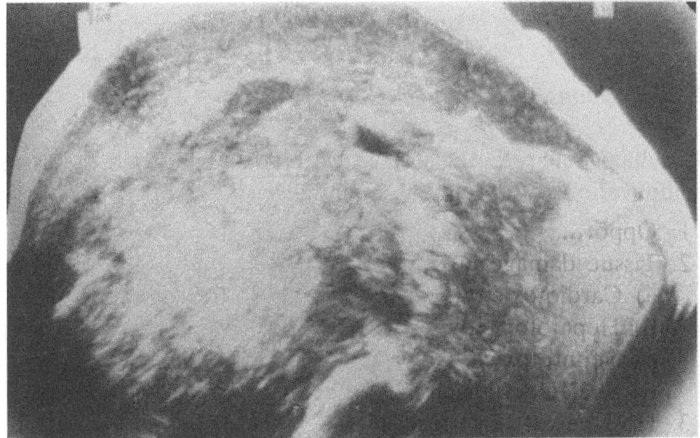

Fig. 5. Neuroblastoma. Transverse sonar scan of epigastrium showing huge irregularly echogenic circular mass displacing liver anteriorly and echofree IVC anteriorly and to the left

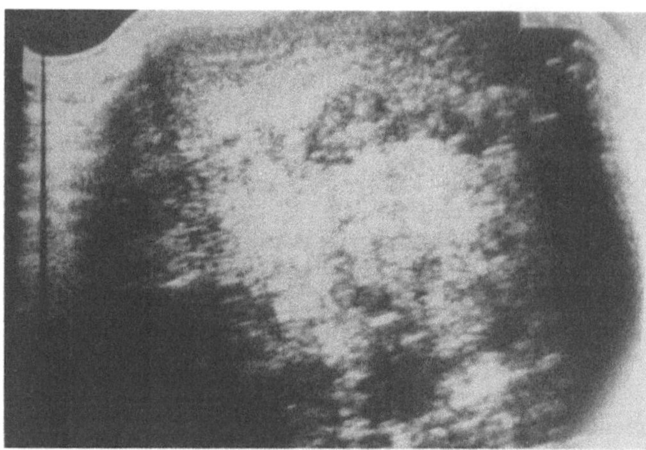

Fig. 6. Neuroblastoma. Longitudinal sonar scan through right lobe of liver showing it displaced anteriorly and superiorly by huge irregularly echogenic circular mass (same child as Fig. 5)

Table 2. UK clinical trial recommendations on follow-up chest x-rays in the first year after diagnosis

Tumour	Recommended interval (weeks)
Yolk-sac	4
Osteogenic sarcoma (first 6 months)	4
Nephroblastoma	6
Non-Hodgkin's lymphoma	6
Osteogenic sarcoma (second 6 months)	6
Rhabdomyosarcoma	8
Ewing's sarcoma	12
Malignant brain tumours	12
Neuroblastoma	16

Complications of Treatment

The diagnostic radiologist may usefully contribute to the assessment of several important complications of treatment, namely:

1. Opportunistic infections.
2. Tissue damage attributable to therapeutic agents:
    a) Cardiotoxicity;
    b) Hepatotoxicity;
    c) Nephrotoxicity;
    d) Skeletal changes.
3. Host versus graft disease.

X-rays are useful in confirming and monitoring opportunistic pneumonitis. Radiographs may help to indicate the optimum site for percutaneous lung biopsy or bronchial brush

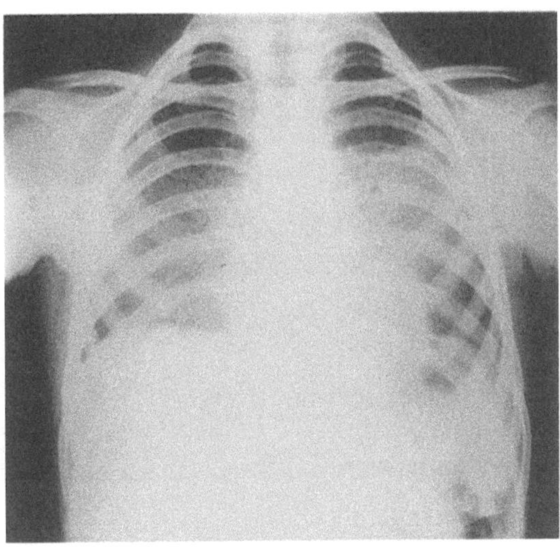

Fig. 7. Opportunistic pneumonitis. Diffuse veiling of lower two-thirds of lung fields with air bronchogram in girl being treated for non-Hodgkin's lymphoma. Proven to be *Pneumocystis carinii* infection

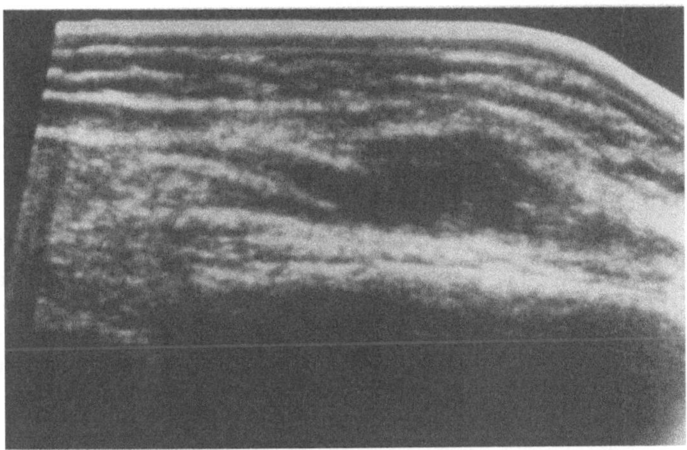

Fig. 8. Quadriceps abscess. Longitudinal sonar scan of right thigh showing localised relatively echofree abscess in quadriceps muscle anterior to femoral shaft. Boy with proven septicaemia during treatment for acute myeloid leukaemia

biopsy where "blind" empirical antibiotic therapy has failed to produce a response. Radiological features are not organism-specific. Most involve x-ray changes (Fig. 7) which are more suggestive of neonatal ideopathic respiratory distress syndrome (extensive air bronchogram or alternating areas of focal collapse and overinflation) than of respiratory infection in children not immunosuppressed (Sweet and Willoughby 1977). Ultrasound may demonstrate abscess formation associated with septicaemia within the abdomen or in soft tissues (Fig. 8).
Echocardiography is the best method for monitoring cardiotoxicity from adriamycin therapy; so a preliminary base line assessment of left ventricular function should be

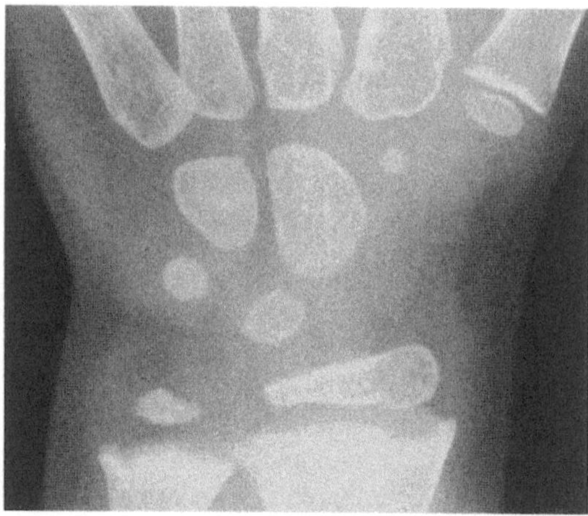

Fig. 9. Methotrexate osteopathy. Wrist showing irregular dense radial and ulnar metaphyses, attributable to minor infractions in boy with wrist pain after prolonged chemotherapy

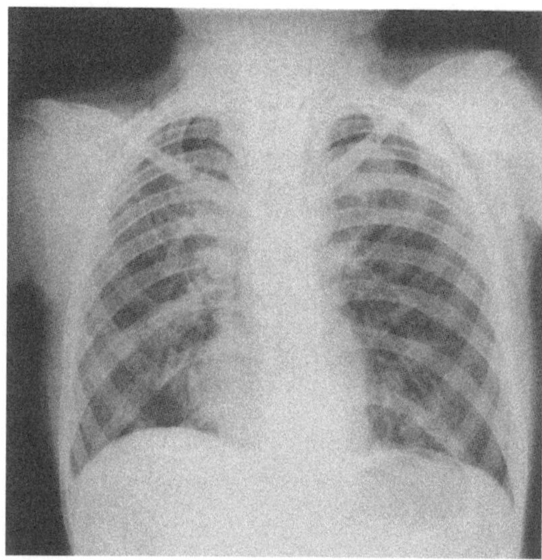

Fig. 10. HVGD pneumonitis. Destructive emphysema affecting both lung fields with bilateral apical pneumothoraces, pneumomediastinum with air tracking up into neck and over lateral chest wall in girl who had had marrow transplant

undertaken before the course of cytotoxic chemotherapy starts and be continued at 4-week intervals.

Fatty changes in the liver can occasionally be demonstrated by increased radiolucency on plain radiography, but the use of sonography to demonstrate changes in tissue characteristics has been found to be a more sensitive method of assessment. Computed tomography may offer similar results.

Isotope investigation of impairment of renal function provides the most sensitive assessment of nephrotoxicity. Cyclophosphamide cystitis may be well demonstrated by intravenous urography or cystography; it may produce severe changes with "thumb printing" sufficiently gross as to mimic the appearance of a rhabdomyosarcoma of the bladder.

Minor trauma in the presence of osteoporosis attributable to therapeutic agents such as steroids and methotrexate may be indistinguishable from metastatic deposits, whether conventional x-rays or isotopes are used (Fig. 9).

Host versus graft disease after bone marrow transplantation may involve the lungs, resulting in progressive destructive emphysema (Fig. 10) which may be complicated by opportunistic infection (Khouri et al. 1979). Liver damage may be monitored by ultrasound or computed tomography as already described.

Follow up After Treatment

After completion of successful treatment diagnostic investigations using ionising radiations are best reserved for suspected local recurrence or metastases and for the assessment of any long term complications of treatment.

Intrathoracic primary tumours or other tumours likely to metastasise to the lungs should be reviewed by simple chest radiography using postero-anterior, lateral and penetrated films. If negative, routine radiography may be followed by whole lung tomography and finally computed tomography if there is strong clinical suspicion of recurrence or metastases.

Ultrasound examination of the contralateral kidney is now to be preferred to frequently repeated intravenous urography in children who have been treated for nephroblastoma as first method of excluding a second renal tumour. If sonar is abnormal, then intravenous urography may be repeated.

In yolk-sac tumours the promising reports of follow-up using labelled radiopharmaceuticals point the way to advances in the follow-up of patients with rising alphafetoprotein levels which indicate recurrent or metastatic disease (Halsall et al. 1981). Future development along similar lines to find other tumour markers will have important implications for the assessment and monitoring of children with malignant disease when more radiopharmaceuticals providing specific labelling become available.

Bone pain calls for skeletal survey using radioisotopes followed by simple radiography of suspicious areas to confirm destruction or pathological fractures attributable to osteoporosis resulting from chemotherapy or radiotherapy.

Bone age estimations (Tanner et al. 1975) are useful in predicting adult height after radiotherapy for intracranial tumours. Also, bone age estimations after treatment of children with leukaemia have produced reassuring information that although growth ceases during treatment it later restarts and resumes along the lower centile (Griffen and Wadsworth 1980).

One problem presented to diagnostic radiologists which could be solved by those responsible for preparation of clinical trial protocols is that of artefacts attributable to metallic clips. Their use on cerebral blood vessels or within the abdomen, as advocated to designate areas of suspicion in the tumour bed on removal of Wilms' tumours for example, causes confusion on both ultrasound and computed tomography, possibly masking locally recurrent disease.

References

1. Appell RC, Brandeis WE, Georgi P, Van Kakk G, Bolkenns M, Ludwig R, Opperman NC, Willich E (1982) Radiographic and scintigraphic appearances of bone-metastasising Wilms' tumour: problems in confirming diagnosis. Ann Radiol 25:14–18
2. Blackledge G, Mamtora H, Crowther D, Isherwood I, Best JJK (1981) The role of abdominal computed tomography in lymphoma following treatment. Br J Radiol 54:955–960

3. Carty H (1982) Personal communication
4. Cohen M, Slabaugh R, Smith JA (1982) Unusual non-metastatic nodules in lungs of children with cancer. Clin Radiol 33:57–59
5. Danis RK, Wolverson MK, Graviss ER, O'Connor DM, Joyce PF, Cradock TV (1979) Pre-operative embolisation of Wilms' tumours. Am J Dis Child 133:503–506
6. Faulkner K, Moores BM (1982) Scattered radiation distribution around computed tomography scanners and the associated radiation hazard to personnel. Br J Radiol 55:70–72
7. Gilday DL, Ash JM, Reilly BJ (1977) Radionuclide skeletal survey for pediatric neoplasms. Radiology 123:399–406
8. Griffen NK, Wadsworth J (1980) Effect of treatment of malignant disease on growth in children. Arch Dis Child 55:600–603
9. Halsall AK, Fairweather DS, Bradwell AR, Blackburn JC, Dykes PW, Howell A, Reeder A, Hine KR (1981) Localisation of malignant germ cell tumours by external scanning after injection of radiolabelled anti-alpha-fetoprotein. Br. Med J 283:942–944
10. Harwood Nash DC (1981) Computed tomography of the pediatric spine: a protocol for the 1980s. Radiol Clin North Am 19:479–494
11. Howman-Giles RB, Gilday DL, Ash JM (1979) Radio-nuclide skeletal survey in neuroblastoma. Radiology 131:497–502
12. Husband JE, Golding SJ (1982) Computed tomography of the body: when should it be used? Br Med J 284:4–8
13. Jaffe MH, White SJ, Silver TM, Heidelberger KP (1981) Wilms' tumour: ultrasonic features, pathological correlation and diagnostic pitfalls. Radiology 140:147–152
14. Khouri NF, Saral R, Armstrong EM, Tutschka PH, Santos GW, Beschorner WE, Siegelman SS (1979) Pulmonary interstitial changes following bone marrow transplantation. Radiology 133:587–592
15. Kuhns LR (1981) Computed tomography of the retroperitoneum in children. Radiol Clin North Am 19:495–501
16. Laurin S, Forsberg L, Johansson A, Jorulf H (1981) Comparative study of angiography, computerised tomography and ultrasound in abdominal tumors of children. Ann Radiol 24:83–90
17. Resjo IM, Harwood-Nash DC, Fitz CR (1979) Computed tomographic metrizamide myelography (CTMM) in intraspinal and paraspinal neoplasms in infants and children. Am J Roentgenol 132:367–372
18. Slovis TL, Philippart MD, Cushing B, Lakshmi D, Perlmutter AD, Reed JO, Wilner HI, Kroovand RL, Farooki ZQ (1981) Evaluation of IVC by sonography and venography in children with renal and hepatic tumours. Radiology 140:767–772
19. Smoger BR, Rosenberg HK, Koss J, Raney R, Belasco BJ, Large P, Arger P (1982) Search for pulmonary metastases in paediatric patients. CT versus conventional radiography. Ann Radiol 25:47–53
20. Sweet EM, Willoughby MLN (1977) Chest x-ray findings in immunosuppressed children presenting with dyspnoea. Ann Radiol 20:71–77
21. Sweet EM, Willoughby MLN (1980) Radiological bone changes in T-cell and "common" ALL of childhood. Br Med J 280:367–368
22. Tanner JM, Whitehouse RH, Marshall WA, Healy MJR, Goldstein H (1975) Assessment of skeletal maturity and prediction of adult height (TW 2 method). Academic Press, London New York San Francisco
23. Tschappeler H, Vock P (1982) Computed tomography and bone tumours in children. Ann Radiol 25:19–24

Acute Lymphoblastic Leukaemia: Achievements and Prospects

R. M. Hardisty

Department for Haematology and Oncology, Institute of Child Health,
The Hospital for Sick Children, Great Ormond Street, London WC1N 1EH, United Kingdom

Introduction

The last major improvement in the outlook for children with acute lymphoblastic leukaemia (ALL) took place around the late 1960s and early 1970s, with the more or less simultaneous introduction of early prophylactic treatment of the central nervous system (CNS) and continuing combination chemotherapy. Since that time, although detailed examination of all aspects of treatment has led to minor advances, there has been no further great stride forward, and treatment remains eventually unsuccessful in about half of all such patients. Meanwhile, however, real advances have been made in the classification of the acute leukaemias, and the prognostic significance of various presenting features has been more closely defined. This new knowledge has influenced the design of therapeutic trials, but it remains to be seen whether prognostic differences can be overcome by the use of more aggressive approaches to the less favourable groups.

Classification

The use of a combination of immunological, biochemical, cytogenetic and morphological techniques has led not only to more precise distinction of different types of acute leukaemia one from another, but also to a better understanding of their pathogenesis in relation to normal stem-cell differentiation and to other lymphoproliferative disorders. The best established morphological classification, which has received wide acceptance, is that of the French-American-British (FAB) group, which recognises three types of lymphoblastic (L1−3) and six types of acute myeloid (M1−6) leukaemia, based on Romanovsky and cytochemical staining (Bennett et al. 1976, 1981).

The original basis of immunological classification of ALL was into T-ALL, B-ALL and non-T, non-B ALL, according to the presence or absence of surface characteristics of these two lymphocyte lines on the leukaemic blast cells. About 85% of childhood ALL falls into the last group, and in the great majority of such cases the blast cells carry the common-ALL (c-ALL) antigen (Greaves et al. 1975) on their surface. This antigen now appears to be a characteristic of early B lymphoblasts, and perhaps about one-third of patients with c-ALL also have immunoglobulin chains in their blast-cell cytoplasm, from which they may be classified as pre-B-ALL (Vogler et al. 1978, Greaves et al. 1979). Surface immunoglobulin, a characteristic of mature B cells, is found in B-ALL, the rarest subclass, which accounts for only 1%−2% of all ALL. T-ALL, characterised by formation of rosettes with papainised sheep erythrocytes (E-rosettes) or the presence of T-cell antigens on the cell surface, comprises 15%−20%, and can be further subdivided into T and pre-T varieties

Recent Results in Cancer Research. Vol. 88
© Springer-Verlag Berlin · Heidelberg 1983

(Thiel et al. 1980). The increasing use of monoclonal antibodies, particularly of the T-cell series, will surely lead to further subclassification, and perhaps to better standardisation of results and nomenclature. These immunological techniques, together with the use of biochemical markers such as terminal deoxynucleotidyl transferase (TdT) and hexosaminidase I, have so far proved of greater value for the light they throw on leukaemogenic mechanisms (Greaves 1981) than in relation to treatment and prognosis.

The most important aspect so far of the cytogenetic classification of ALL is the recognition that a proportion of such cases carry the Philadelphia (Ph') chromosome in their leukaemic cells: only about 1%−2% of childhood cases (Chessells et al. 1979), but a higher proportion of adults (Bloomfield et al. 1977). This observation is not only of great theoretical interest in relation to bone marrow ontogeny, but also of prognostic importance, since such patients usually respond poorly to treatment. Another specific cytogenetic marker is the 14q+ abnormality seen in B-cell lymphomas and in B-ALL. This is the only variety of ALL in which the immunological and morphological classifications correlate: L3 leukaemia is the morphological description of B-ALL, but the L1/L2 distinction is unrelated to the immunological subtype.

Prognostic Factors

Certain presenting clinical and haematological features − notably leucocyte count, organomegaly, age, race and sex − have been recognised for many years as influencing the eventual outcome of treatment in ALL (Hardisty and Till 1968; Miller 1975), and various others have been added subsequently (Table 1). Not all the features listed in Table 1 are of equal weight, and the apparent prognostic significance of many of them has varied widely from one series of patients to another. None would dispute, however, that the leucocyte count remains the best indicator of prognosis, and stratification of patients into risk groups for therapeutic purposes has usually depended solely or chiefly on this. Many of the factors are interdependent, so that their individual prognostic significance may be hard to assess: T-ALL, for example, is relatively common in older boys and is usually associated with a high leucocyte count (Graeves et al. 1981); early CNS involvement and slowness to remit are common features of B-ALL (L3); and a high leucocyte count often coexists with prominent hepatosplenomegaly. Other features, however, appear to exert an independent effect, and several groups of investigators (Miller et al. 1980, 1981; Henze et al. 1981; Palmer et al. 1980) have devised multifactorial prognostic scoring systems, using multiple regression analysis, to take account of this. It must be stressed, of course, that treatment remains the most important determinant of prognosis, and that the relative importance of the various presenting features will differ from one therapeutic regime to another. It should

Table 1. ALL: adverse prognostic features

High white blood cell (WBC) count	Hepatosplenomegaly
L2 or L3 (FAB)	Male gender
Age < 2 or > 8	Pseudodiploidy
Low IG	Slowness to remit
Low PAS score	Early CNS disease
High Hb	Black race
T- or B-ALL	

be the aim of any new treatment protocol to reduce the prognostic significance of all these clinical and haematological features by improving the results obtained in the most adverse group to the level of those achieved in the most favourable.

The effect of many of these adverse features, including leucocyte count, is confined to the first 2−3 years after diagnosis (Sather et al. 1981): for example, although the relapse rate during this time increases with the initial leucocyte count, the risk of subsequent relapse in patients with high counts who have survived this period in continuous remission is no greater than in those with low counts at diagnosis. A notable exception to this pattern is shown in the effect of sex. No difference emerges during the first 2−3 years, but boys then tend to continue to relapse − in the bone marrow as well as the testis − for longer than girls before a plateau is reached. Possible explanations for this difference, which varies greatly in degree from one trial to another, and was particularly marked in the MRC UKALL II trials (Medical Research Council 1978), are considered further below.

The prognostic significance of chromosomal classification of the blast cells has been shown to be largely independent of that of age, sex and leucocyte count. While pseudodiploidy carries an adverse prognosis, hyperdiploidy and hypodiploidy both appear to be associated with greater duration of remission and longer survival than a normal karyotype (Secker-Walker et al. 1978, 1982). The adverse effect of pseudodiploidy is only partly attributable to the inclusion of cases with specific marker chromosomes, notably the Ph′ chromosome, in this category.

Principles of Primary Treatment

Remission Induction

The induction of a complete remission is the first aim of treatment and presents no great difficulty in most cases of childhood ALL. The combination of vincristine and prednisolone is successful in about 90% of patients (Hardisty et al. 1969; Medical Research Council 1971) and the addition of L-asparaginase may improve the remission rate still further (Ortega et al. 1977). Expert supportive care is essential at this stage, particularly in patients with very high blast cell counts, in order to prevent avoidable complications such as uric acid nephropathy, electrolyte disturbances and serious haemorrhage and infection. The risk of the last two of these is of appreciably less duration than in AML, however, since the platelet and neutrophil counts usually begin to recover within the first couple of weeks.

Failure to remit within 3−4 weeks calls for a reappraisal of the diagnosis. B-ALL, unclassified ("null") ALL and Ph′-positive ALL are all relatively resistant to remission induction, and the possibility that the patient has a poorly differentiated AML must also be considered. Patients with T-ALL, although they are at high risk of early relapse, usually enter their initial remission rapidly (Chessells et al. 1977).

Prevention of Bone Marrow Relapse

Haematological relapse remains the chief barrier to successful treatment of ALL. Although second remissions can usually be achieved, the ultimate prognosis for relapsed patients is poor, and very long-term survivals are largely confined to those who have never relapsed (Hardisty et al. 1981). Many different types of continuing combination chemotherapy have been used in the attempt to eradicate residual cells from the bone marrow after induction of remission, and so to prevent relapse. Most have been based on methotrexate and 6-mercaptopurine, with the addition of various other drugs. Individual protocols have varied from intermittent short intensive courses to continuous maintenance therapy on which occasional consolidation courses of other drugs are superimposed. There is now fairly wide agreement that continuation of this phase of treatment for more than 2–3 years carries no advantage (George et al. 1979; Mandelli et al. 1980; Medical Research Council 1982). It appears also that there is little to choose between the various types of combination chemotherapy which have been employed. Evidence is accumulating, however, to suggest that early intensification of therapy, whether by the use of additional drugs during remission induction, by a period of further intensive consolidation soon after remission has been achieved, or by both, may be the most effective way of preventing bone marrow relapse (Simone 1976). The most encouraging results of this approach so far reported are those of the West German group (Henze et al. 1981).

They used a seven-drug induction regime, followed in "high-risk" patients by a further 6-week course of intensive consolidation, and have apparently achieved a 3-year complete remission rate of 75% in their "high-risk" group, so eliminating the effect of adverse prognostic features. Further follow-up will be necessary before these results can be fully assessed, but they justify further randomised trials of similar regimes, to determine which are the essential components and which patients can benefit from such treatment.

Prevention of Central Nervous System Relapse

Since the early trials of radiotherapy and intrathecal methotrexate by Pinkel and his colleagues (for review, see Hustu and Aur 1978), CNS prophylaxis has been an essential part of the management of ALL in childhood. In the MRC'S UKALL series of trials, a total dose of 2,400 cGy to the cranium has been combined with either the same dose to the spinal axis, intrathecal methotrexate alone or a combination of intrathecal methotrexate with a spinal dose of 1,000 cGy. The last of these regimes has proved marginally more effective than the second, while radiotherapy alone, without methotrexate, was not only the least successful in preventing CNS relapse, but in "poor-risk" patients was also associated with the highest bone marrow relapse rate (Hardisty 1982).

The possibly deleterious effect of CNS irradiation on learning ability, particularly in young children (Eiser 1978, 1980), as well as the risk of other long-term toxic effects, led the American Children's Cancer Study Group to compare 1,800 cGy with 2,400 cGy for either cranial or craniospinal irradiation (Nesbit et al. 1981b). They found that the lower dose was equally effective, and it has now been adopted by the MRC Working Party. Other groups have used methotrexate without radiotherapy for CNS prophylaxis, either intrathecally or in moderately high dose intravenously (Haghbin 1976; Freeman et al. 1977), but most now favour some combination of radiation and chemotherapy.

Death and Morbidity During Complete Remission

Infections present a serious risk to children in remission on chemotherapy; of 168 children with ALL treated at the Hospital for Sick Children in London between 1973 and 1977, 76 (45%) required at least one admission to hospital on account of infection, and 13 (8%) died in remission (Ninane and Chessells 1981). The most important infections are listed in

Table 2. Serious infections during remission

Measles:	Pneumonia Encephalitis	*Pneumocystis carinii:*	Pneumonia
Varicella zoster:	Dissemination Encephalitis	*Cytomegalovirus*	Gram-negative septicaemia

Table 2. Measles is a particular hazard in Britain, on account of the poor rate of acceptance of measles vaccination. The incidence of pneumocystis pneumonia is related to the degree of immunosuppression caused by the treatment (Hughes et al. 1975); it is less common in patients receiving intermittent therapy, whose lymphocyte counts are less depressed than those of patients on continuous treatment (Rapson et al. 1980). It can largely be prevented by the use of prophylactic cotrimoxazole (Hughes et al. 1977). Specific *varicella/zoster* immunoglobulin can prevent or modify chickenpox if given soon after contact, and active immunisation with varicella vaccine may prove effective (Ha et al. 1980). Acyclovir is also helpful in the treatment of herpes-virus infections (Selby et al. 1979). Gram-negative septicaemia is a hazard in neutropenic patients, while the virus infections are associated with lymphocyte depletion. Avoidance of all these infective complications demands a high degree of awareness of risk factors, with consequent early diagnosis and vigorous treatment.

Prevention of Testicular Relapse

The incidence of overt testicular infiltration varies widely between reported series. The complication occasionally occurs during treatment, particularly in boys with adverse prognostic features. Its main incidence is during the first year after stopping chemotherapy (Medical Research Council 1978; Nesbit et al. 1980), when it is often shortly followed by bone marrow relapse. There has been much discussion as to whether the testis acts as a sanctuary in which the leukaemic cells are partially protected from the action of the chemotherapeutic agents, and from which they reseed the bone marrow, or whether testicular relapse merely reflects a more generalised dissemination of the disease. If the former is correct, then early "prophylactic" irradiation of the testes, at the cost of permanent sterilisation, might be expected to diminish the incidence of late bone marrow relapse as well as overt testicular infiltration. The initial results of a trial of early testicular irradiation in boys with adverse prognostic features, however, suggest that it has no effect on the bone marrow relapse rate, although it greatly reduces the incidence of overt testicular infiltration (Medical Research Council, unpublished). In practice, many groups, including the MRC Working Party, now adopt a policy of performing bilateral wedge biopsy of the testes before stopping chemotherapy. Patients with microscopic infiltration receive bilateral radiotherapy (2,400 cGy), and their systemic chemotherapy is continued (see below). .

Chronic Sequelae of Treatment

Besides the acute infective complications of treatment discussed above, its long-term consequences become increasingly important as more children survive their acute leukaemia into adult life. These include post-infective complications, particularly after measles, neurological complications of radiotherapy and chemotherapy — particularly in patients who have required further treatment for a CNS relapse —, interference with intellectual development, with growth or with fertility, liver damage and fibrosis, and finally the risk of second neoplasms. Although the effects on growth and learning ability are usually small, and the other long-term complications fortunately rare, these constraints on the design of therapeutic regimes must not be underestimated.

Treatment After Relapse

Bone Marrow Relapse

Although second remissions can be readily achieved in most patients, the subsequent prognosis for cure is very poor, especially for those who relapse while still on chemotherapy (Cornbleet and Chessells 1978; Ekert et al. 1979). Relapses occurring a year or more after stopping chemotherapy are more likely to be followed by a prolonged second remission (Chessells and Breatnach 1981), but the ultimate prognosis remains much poorer than in previously untreated patients. In children who relapse at or soon after the end of chemotherapy, and who are fortunate enough to have a histocompatible sibling donor, the treatment of choice following the induction of a second remission is now total body irradiation followed by allogeneic bone marrow transplantation (BMT). The same may be true in the case of later relapses, though here a case can be made for a second attempt at eradication of the leukaemia by conventional therapy alone. Johnson et al. (1981) compared the response rate of 24 children transplanted in second or subsequent remission with that of 21 relapsed children who received conventional chemotherapy. Nine of the transplanted group remained in continuous complete remission for 17−55 months after BMT, but only one of the chemotherapy group was still in remission at 20 months.

Central Nervous System Relapse

This still occurs in 5%−10% of children despite prophylaxis. There is seldom any difficulty in clearing leukaemic cells from the cerebrospinal fluid (CSF) with intrathecal methotrexate; however, eradication of the perivascular infiltrates beneath the meninges is harder to achieve, and recurrences are common. Craniospinal irradiation is the treatment of choice, following the initial course of methotrexate, in patients who have not been previously irradiated (Willoughby 1976). It has also sometimes proved effective in the treatment of patients relapsing some years after prophylactic cranial irradiation (Wells et al. 1980). An alternative approach is the use of repeated intrathecal methotrexate every 4−6 weeks for at least 2 years, either by the lumbar route or via an intraventricular reservoir (Gribbin et al. 1977). Both reirradiation and intraventricular chemotherapy carry a risk of leucoencephalopathy (Kay et al. 1972; Rubinstein et al. 1975), and the two forms of treatment must not be combined.

Although CNS relapse is compatible with prolonged bone marrow remission, the risk of haematological relapse remains high in such patients (Gribbin et al. 1977; Nesbit et al. 1981a); therefore a course of systemic induction therapy followed by a further 2−3 years of continuing combination chemotherapy is therefore to be recommended.

Testicular Relapse

Leukaemic infiltration of the testes, whether detected microscopically at biopsy or diagnosed clinically, can usually be effectively eradicated by a radiation dose of 2,500 cGy to both testes and spermatic cords (Sullivan et al. 1980). In view of the high risk of subsequent bone marrow relapse, systemic chemotherapy should also be reinstituted and continued for 2 years; a further short course of prophylactic intrathecal methotrexate is also advisable. Chessells (1982) observed no subsequent relapses in ten boys treated in this way after an isolated testicular relapse; all but one of these boys had come to the end of a further 2 years' chemotherapy.

Possible Future Developments

Where should we now be looking for further therapeutic advances? New cytotoxic drugs and drug combinations are constantly under trial, but it remains disappointingly true that the four most valuable drugs — vincristine, prednisolone, mercaptopurine and metho-trexate — have all been available for over 20 years. The addition of the more modern drugs has made little difference yet to the outlook for children with ALL. Amongst those which hold out some promise are 4'-(9-acridimylamino-methanesulphon-m-aniside) (m-AMSA) (Rivera et al. 1980) and, for T-ALL in particular, the adenosine deaminase inhibitor 2-deoxycoformycin (Prentice et al. 1980, 1981).

A more specific attack on residual leukaemic cells might theoretically be mounted by means of leukaemia-specific antibodies, either by relying on their own cytotoxicity or by conjugating them with toxins such as ricin. Such an approach has been used to deplete the patient's marrow of leukaemic cells in vitro, prior to reinjecting it after intensive chemotherapy and irradiation (Netzel et al. 1980) and might even be applicable in vivo (Ritz and Schlossman 1982). Unfortunately, however, there is no good evidence than any of the antibodies so far produced against leukaemic cells are in fact leukaemia-specific. The c-ALL-associated antigen has been identified on a population of normal lymphoid precursors (Greaves et al. 1980), so that the use of the corresponding antibody in this way might be expected to jeopardise the reconstitution of normal marrow elements. Similar objections probably apply to the therapeutic use of antibodies directed against B-ALL and T-ALL cells.

Perhaps the best grounds for optimism in the near future will be provided by improvements in bone marrow transplantation. Because of the need for an HLA-indentical sibling donor, this form of treatment is only available for about one-third of patients at present, but if the major problem of graft-versus-host disease can be overcome, whether by enrichment of stem cells in the donor marrow at the expense of immunocompetent T cells or by improved chemotherapy after transplantation, it may become possible to transplant patients across the histocompatibility barrier.

While multicentre trials have contributed largely — and will surely continue to contribute — to improvements in treatment of ALL, many of the more intractable problems with which we are now faced will need the particular expertise and facilities of specialised centres for their solution. Whatever our therapeutic aims in the future, the careful design of controlled clinical trials must remain a paramount consideration.

R. M. Hardisty

References

1. Bennett JM, Catovsky D, Daniel MT, Flandrin G, Galton DAG, Gralnick HR, Sultan C (1976) Proposals for the classification of the acute leukaemias. Br J Haematol 33: 451–458

2. Bennett JM, Catovsky D, Daniel MT, Flandrin G, Galton DAG, Gralnick HR, Sultan C, The French-American-British (FAB) Cooperative Group (1981) The morphological classification of acute lymphoblastic leukaemia: concordance among observers and clinical correlations. Br J Haematol 47: 553–561

3. Bloomfield CD, Peterson LC, Yunis JJ, Brunning RD (1977) The Philadelphia chromosome (Ph') in adults presenting with acute leukaemia: a comparison of Ph'+ and Ph'− patients. Br J Haematol 36: 347–358

4. Chessells JM (1982) Some aspects of treatment of childhood leukaemia. In: Valman HB (ed) Topics in paediatrics 3. Recent advances in paediatric therapeutics. Pitman, London, pp 129–138

5. Chessells JM, Breatnach F (1981) Late marrow relapses in childhood acute lymphoblastic leukaemia. Br Med J 283: 649–751

6. Chessells JM, Hardisty RM, Rapson NT, Greaves MF (1977) Acute lymphoblastic leukaemia in children: classification and prognosis. Lancet 2: 1307–1309

7. Chessells JM, Janossy G, Lawler SD, Secker-Walker LM (1979) The Ph' chromosome in childhood leukaemia. Br J Haematol 41: 25–41

8. Cornbleet MA, Chessells JM (1978) Bone-marrow relapse in acute lymphoblastic leukaemia in childhood. Br Med J 2: 104–106

9. Eiser C (1978) Intellectual abilities among survivors of childhood leukaemia as a function of CNS irradiation. Arch Dis Child 53: 391–395

10. Eiser C (1980) Effects of chronic illness on intellectual development. A comparison of normal children with those treated for childhood leukaemia and solid tumours. Arch Dis Child 55: 766–770

11. Ekert H, Ellis WM, Waters KD, Matthews RM (1979) Poor outlook for childhood acute lymphoblastic leukaemia with relapse. Med J Aust 2: 224–226

12. Freeman AI, Wang JJ, Sinks LF (1977) High dose methotrexate in acute lymphocytic leukemia. Cancer Treat Rep 61: 727–731

13. George SL, Aur RJA, Mauer AM, Simone JV (1979) A reappraisal of the results of stopping therapy in childhood leukemia. New Engl J Med 300: 269–273

14. Greaves MF (1981) Biology of acute lymphoblastic leukaemia. Leukaemia Research Fund. 16th Annual Guest Lecture

15. Greaves MF, Brown G, Rapson NT, Lister TA (1975) Antisera to acute lymphoblastic leukaemia cells. Clin Immunol Immunopathol 4: 67–84

16. Greaves MF, Verbi W, Vogler L, Cooper M, Ellis R, Ganeshaguru K, Hoffbrand V, Janossy G, Bollum FJ (1979) Antigenic and enzymatic phenotypes of the pre-B subclass of acute lymphoblastic leukaemia. Leukaemia Res 3: 353–362

17. Greaves MF, Delia D, Janossy G, Rapson N, Chessells J, Woods M, Prentice G (1980) Acute lymphoblastic leukaemia associated antigen. IV. Expression on non-leukaemic 'lymphoid' cells. Leuk Res 4: 15–32

18. Greaves MF, Janossy G, Peto J, Kay HEM (1981) Immunologically defined subclasses of acute lymphoblastic leukaemia in children: their relationship to presentation features and prognosis. Br J Haematol 48: 179–197

19. Gribbin MA, Hardisty RM, Chessells JM (1977) Long-term control of central nervous system leukaemia. Arch Dis Child 52: 673–678

20. Ha K, Baba K, Ikeda T, Nishida M, Yabuuchi H, Takahashi M (1980) Application of live varicella vaccine to children with acute leukemia or other malignancies without suspension of anticancer therapy. Pediatrics 65: 346–350

21. Haghbin M (1976) Chemotherapy of acute lymphoblastic leukemia in children. Am J Hematol 1: 201–209

22. Hardisty RM (1982) Prophylaxis of central-nervous-system leukaemia: British experience, 1970–80. Proceedings of the International Pediatric Oncology Conference, Rome, October 1981, pp 140–143
23. Hardisty RM, Till MM (1968) Acute leukaemia 1959–1964: factors affecting prognosis. Arch Dis Child 43: 107–115
24. Hardisty RM, McElwain TJ, Darby CW (1969) Vincristine and prednisolone for the induction of remission in acute childhood leukaemia. Br Med J 2: 662–665
25. Hardisty RM, Till MM, Peto J (1981) Acute lymphoblastic leukaemia: four-year survivals old and new. J Clin Pathol 34: 249–253
26. Henze G, Langermann H-J, Ritter J, Schellong G. Riehm H-J (1981) Treatment strategy for different risk groups in childhood acute lymphoblastic leukaemia. A report from the BFM Study Group. In: Neth R, Gollo RC, Hofschneider PH, Monnweiler K (eds) Modern trends in human leukaemia IV. Springer-Verlag, Heidelberg, pp 87–93
27. Hughes WT, Feldman S, Aur RJA, Verzosa MS, Hustu HO, Simone JV (1975) Intensity of immunosuppressive therapy and the incidence of *Pneumocystis carinii* pneumonitis. Cancer 36: 2004–2009
28. Hughes WT, Kuhn S, Chaudhary S, Feldman S, Verzosa M, Aur RJA, Pratt C, George SL (1977) Successful chemo-prophylaxis for *Pneumocystis carinii* pneumonitis. New Engl J Med 297: 1419–1426
29. Hustu HO, Aur RJA (1978) Extramedullary leukaemia. Clin Haematol 7: 313–337
30. Johnson FL, Thomas ED, Clark BS, Chard RL, Hartmann JR, Storb R (1981) A comparison of marrow transplantation with chemotherapy for children with acute lymphoblastic leukaemia in second or subsequent remission. N Engl J Med 305: 846–851
31. Kay HEM, Knapton PJ, O'Sullivan JP, Wells DG, Harris DG, Harris RF, Innes EM, Stuart J, Schwartz FCM, Thompson EN (1972) Encephalopathy in acute leukaemia associated with methotrexate therapy. Arch Dis Child 47: 344–354
32. Mandelli F, Amadori S, Rajnoldi AC, di Montezemolo LC, Madon E, Masera G, Meloni G, Pacilli L, Paolucci G, Pastore G, Rosito P, Uderzo C, Vecchi V (1980) Discontinuing therapy in childhood acute lymphocytic leukaemia. Cancer 46: 1319–1323
33. Medical Research Council (1971) Treatment of acute lymphoblastic leukaemia. Comparison of immunotherapy (B.C.G), intermittent methotrexate, and no therapy after a two-month intensive cytotoxic regimen. Br Med J 4: 189–194
34. Medical Research Council (1978) Testicular disease in acute lymphoblastic leukaemia in childhood. Br Med J 1: 334–338
35. Medical Research Council (1982) Duration of chemotherapy in childhood acute lymphoblastic leukemia (ALL). Med Pediatr Oncol (in press)
36. Miller DR (1975) Prognostic factors in childhood leukemia. J Pediatr 87: 672–676
37. Miller DR, Leikin S, Albo V, Vitale L, Sather H, Coccia P, Nesbit M, Karon M, Hammond D (1980) Use of prognostic factors in improving the design and efficiency of clinical trials in childhood leukemia: Children's Cancer Study Group report. Cancer treat Rep 64: 381–392
38. Miller DR, Leikin S, Albo V, Sather H, Hammond D (1981) Prognostic importance of morphology (FAB classification) in childhood acute lymphoblastic leukaemia (ALL). Br J Haematol 48: 199–206
39. Nesbit ME, Robison LL, Ortega JA, Sather HN, Donaldson M, Hammond D (1980) Testicular relapse in childhood acute lymphoblastic leukemia: association with pretreatment, patient characteristics and treatment. Cancer 45: 2009–2016
40. Nesbit ME, D'Angio GJ, Sather HN, Robison LL, Ortega J, Donaldson M, Hammond GD (1981a) Effect of isolated central nervous system leukaemia on bone marrow remission and survival in childhood acute lymphoblastic leukaemia: association with pretreatment, patient characteristics and treatment. Lancet 1: 1386–1389
41. Nesbit ME, Sather HN, Robison LL, Ortega J, Littman PS, D'Angio GJ, Hammond GD (1981b) Presymptomatic central nervous system therapy in previously untreated childhood acute lymphoblastic leukaemia: comparison of 1,800 rad and 2,400 rad. Lancet 1: 461–466

42. Netzel B, Haas RJ, Rodt H, Kolb HJ, Thierfelder S (1980) Immunological conditioning of bone marrow for autotransplantation in childhood acute lymphoblastic leukaemia. Lancet 1:1330–1332
43. Ninane J, Chessells JM (1981) Serious infections during continuing treatment of acute lymphoblastic leukaemia. Arch Dis Child 56:841–844
44. Ortega JA, Nesbit ME, Donaldson MH, Hittle RE, Weiner J, Karon M, Hammond D (1977) L-asparaginase, vincristine and prednisone for induction of first remission in acute lymphocytic leukaemia. Cancer Res 37:535–540
45. Palmer MK, Hann I, Jones PM, Evans DIK (1980) A score at diagnosis for predicting length of remission in childhood lymphoblastic leukaemia. Br J Cancer 42:841–849
46. Prentice HG, Smyth JF, Ganeshaguru K, Wonke B, Bradstock KF, Janossy G, Goldstone AH, Hoffbrand AV (1980) Remission induction with adenosine-deaminase inhibitor 2'-deoxycoformycin in thylymphoblastic leukaemia. Lancet 2:170–172
47. Prentice HG, Russell NH, Lee N, Ganeshaguru K, Blacklock H, Piga A, Smyth JF, Hoffbrand AV (1981) Therapeutic selectivity of and prediction of response to 2'-deoxycoformycin in acute leukaemia. Lancet 2:1250–1253
48. Rapson NT, Cornbleet MA, Chessells JM, Bennett T, Hardisty RM (1980) Immunosuppression and serious infections in children with acute lymphoblastic leukaemia: a comparison of three chemotherapy regimes. Br J Haematol 45:41–52
49. Ritz J, Schlossman SF (1982) Utilization of monoclonal antibodies in the treatment of leukemia and lymphoma. Blood 59:1–11
50. Rivera G, Evans WE, Dahl GV, Yee GC, Pratt CB (1980) Phase 1 clinical and pharmacokinetic study of 4'(9-acridimylamino-methanesulfon-m-aniside) in children with cancer. Cancer Res 40:4250–4253
51. Rubinstein LJ, Herman MM, Long TF, Wilbur JR (1975) Disseminated necrotizing leukoencephalopathy: a complication of treated central nervous system leukemia and lymphoma. Cancer 35:291–305
52. Sather H, Coccia P, Nesbit M, Level C, Hammond D (1981) Disappearance of the predictive value of prognostic variables in childhood acute lymphoblastic leukemia. Cancer 48:370–376
53. Secker-Walker LM, Lawler SD, Hardisty RM (1978) Prognostic implications of chromosome findings in acute lymphoblastic leukaemia at diagnosis. Br Med J 2:1529–1530
54. Secker-Walker LM, Swansbury GJ, Hardisty R, Sallan SE, Garson OM, Sakurai M, Lawler SD (1982) Cytogenetics of acute lympoblastic leukaemia in children as a factor in the prediction of long term survival. Br J Haematol (in press)
55. Selby PJ, Powles RL, Jameson BJ, Kay HEM, Watson JG, Thornton R, Morgenstern G, Clink HM, McElwain TJ, Prentice HG, Corringham R, Ross MG, Hoffbrand AV, Brigden D (1979) Parenteral acyclovir therapy for herpes virus infections in man. Lancet 2:1267–1270
56. Simone JV (1976) Factors that influence remission duration in acute lymphocytic leukaemia. Br J Haematol 32:465–472
57. Sullivan MP, Perez CA, Herson J, Silva-Sousa M, Land V, Dyment PG, Cahn R, Ayala AG (1980) Radiotherapy (2,500 rad) for testicular leukemia. Local control and subsequent clinical events: A South-West Oncology Group study. Cancer 46:508–515
58. Thiel E, Rodt H, Huhn D, Netzel B, Grosse-Wilde H, Ganeshaguru K, Thierfelder S (1980) Multimarker classification of acute lymphoblastic leukemia: evidence for further T sub-groups and evaluation of their clinical significance. Blood 56:759–772
59. Vogler LB, Crist WM, Bockman DE, Pearl ER, Lawton AR, Cooper MD (1978) Pre-B-cell leukemia. A new phenotype of childhood lymphoblastic leukemia. New Engl J Med 298:872–878
60. Wells RJ, Weetman RM, Baehner RL (1980) The impact of isolated central nervous system relapse following initial complete remission in childhood acute lymphocytic leukemia. J Pediatr 97:429–432
61. Willoughby MLN (1976) Treatment of overt meningeal leukaemia in children: results of second MRC meningeal leukaemia trial. Br Med J 1:864–867

The Psychological Sequelae of Childhood Leukaemia*

G. P. Maguire

Department of Psychiatry, University Hospital of South Manchester,
Manchester M20 8LE, United Kingdom

Introduction

The outlook for children suffering from acute lymphoblastic leukaemia has improved
considerably over the last decade. Fifty per cent are expected to survive at least 5 years
while some may eventually be considered "cured". This contrasts sharply with the 1960s
when the disease was invariably fatal. Paradoxically, this change in prognosis has increased
the strain on parents and they have to surmount several hurdles if they are to avoid serious
psychological problems and lead a reasonably normal life.

Coping With Uncertainty

While the clinician can usually provide some indication of the probable outcome in a given
child, it is not possible to make an exact prediction. The parents, therefore, have to come to
terms with the awful uncertainty about their child's future. If the child survives the first 2–3
years of active treatment the parents have to decide whether or not they should take the
risk of deciding that their child is now cured. Their feelings of uncertainty may be
heightened every time they visit the treatment centre, for the examination and
investigations will reveal how the child is progressing. They may worry greatly about the
possible results, especially if they meet parents whose child has relapsed after being on
similar treatment. Attempts to put any worries to the back of their minds may also be
hindered by the increased attention given to leukaemia in childhood by the mass media,
particularly controversies about possible but unproven alternative therapies. Parents have
to find ways of coping with this uncertainty if they are to prevent themselves being
overwhelmed by unremitting worry about the possibility of relapse and death (Comaroff
and Maguire 1981).

Tolerating the Adverse Effects of Treatment

The cytotoxic drugs and radiotherapy which are used to treat childhood leukaemia often
cause unpleasant symptoms. These include nausea, vomiting, tiredness, hair loss, mouth
ulcers and weight gain and may be intense in degree. They may be so unpleasant that the
parents become reluctant to accept further treatment. Some parents experience much

---

* This chapter was possible through the generous financial support of the Leukaemia Research Fund
and the Social Science Research Council

strain because they cannot bear to watch their child suffer yet know that he or she will die if treatment stops. Treatment involves repeated injections, and children who already have a phobia of needles may find this intolerable. Others find that they develop a conditioned reflex. The mention, sight or smell of the hospital causes them to feel sick or vomit. Teenagers can find the hair loss particularly upsetting. When these adverse effects occur they may upset parents and remind them of the seriousness of their child's illness.

Managing Visits to Hospital

Treatment is usually carried out within a special centre. Consequently, some parents have to travel a considerable distance. They may find it difficult to arrange transport, to geht time off work or to find relatives and friends who are willing to look after any other children. The cost of repeated visiting and time off work may cause financial hardship (Bodkin et al. 1982).

The current emphasis on encouraging parents to be with their child when he or she is in hospital derives from arguments that this will avoid separation anxiety and so prevent behavioural problems. However, the pendulum of change from restricted to open visiting may have swung too far. Parents feel guilty if they are away from the hospital and yet worry about their other children. Lengthy or repeated stays in hospital can result in one or both parents becoming isolated from the rest of their family. They are also at risk from having too litte "time out" from the problem and of becoming too exhausted physically and too drained emotionally.

How to Balance Needs

One of the most difficult issues for parents is how to do all they can to ensure that their child survives while attempting to live a reasonably normal life. Can they trust their child in the hands of a babysitter? Can they go out together without constantly thinking of the sick child and feeling they have no right to enjoy themselves? Parents also have to try to meet each other's needs and those of their other children. Yet they often find that all their attention and energy are being directed toward the sick child and that others are being neglected. While they may realise this they usually feel powerless to resolve the situation.

How to Treat the Child Normally

Parents are commonly advised by the paediatrician to treat their child as normal. How can they, when the child may be dead within a few months? They may say, as one mother did, "How can I possibly still smack him when he is naughty − I cannot bear to think that this could be his last memory of me". Consequently, parents may relax their discipline, and overindulge and overprotect the child.

What Should the Child be Told?

Parents have to decide what to tell the sick child, their other children, relatives and friends about the nature of the illness. Some elect to be open, and this favours the psychological and social adjustment of the familiy in the longer term (Slavin et al. 1982). Others decide to provide a cover story such as "you have a special kind of anaemia". They may then feel under considerable pressure because they are aware that they are living a lie, are worried about the effects of this on their children and others, and feat that the children may have seen through the deception.

Resisting Isolation

When a child suffers an acute illness close relatives and friends usually keep in regular touch with the parents to ask how the child is progressing. They can reasonably predict that the answer will be encouraging and that the illness will soon be over. The situation with a chronic life-threatening illness like leukaemia is very different. Even if the child gets into remission he or she still has to go regularly for treatment and the parent cannot say that the child is cured. Parents usually realise within a few months of diagnosis that many of their close relatives and friends have ceased to ask them about their child's progress and have also stopped seeing or contacting them. Consequently, they become increasingly isolated and separated from their normal sources of support.

This isolation is often intensified by the family's feeling that it has been stigmatised. Death in a child is now a rare event. Parents ask — why us? why our child? why now? They feel they have been singled out for misfortune and may feel extremely bitter. They may also wonder why another less pleasant and well-mannered child was not chosen for this fate. They often feel unclean and worry that the leukaemia could be contagious. Indeed, parents often report that others treat them "as though we had leprosy in the family".

Families also tend to become isolated from their own doctors. Few general practitioners care for many children with leukaemia during their professional lifetime. Moreover, the practitioners are not usually aware of the latest advances in treatment. They may, therefore, feel at a disadvantage when faced with a mother or father who wants to discuss the child's progress and treatment. Doctors may react by seeing less of the family than they would otherwise have done, and may also visit less because of the emotional strain this places on them (Rosser and Maguire 1982). The doctor who brought the child into the world may find it upsetting to face the possibility that this child could soon die. The feeling that it should have been realised earlier that the child had a serious illness may also cause the doctor to avoid the family.

Most families will interpret such avoidance as a lack of interest and concern. They will be inclined to devalue the help of the general practitioner and look increasingly towards the treatment centre for support. However, the treatment centre will assume that the general practitioner, relatives and friends are still providing support. Consequently, families may perceive both the hospital and primary care teams as unhelpful and become even more isolated.

Search for Meaning

Most parents try desperately to search for an explanation as to why their child has contracted leukaemia (Comaroff and Maguire 1981). They will sometimes search extremely hard for such information and be very frustrated and upset when they realise that relatively little is known about the aetiology. Parents are at risk of blaming themselves or some external cause. Such self-blame can become morbid as the following example illustrates: one mother had an argument with her priest a few years before her child became ill. She had wanted to take the contraceptive pill but her priest said that this was against the Church's teaching. She went against his advice and took the pill for a year before deciding together with her husband that they wanted a further child. This child developed leukaemia and the mother became convinced against argument that this was a punishment from God for deceiving the Church. She became extremely depressed and required psychiatric help.

Failure of Parenting

The rarity of death in childhood causes some parents to feel extremely guilty that they have failed to succeed in their task of helping their child achieve adulthood without suffering major physical illness. They may become overwhelmed by feelings of failure and helplessness because they believe that there is little they can do to remedy the situation. These are all formidable hurdles and it should not be surprising that some families fail to surmount them and develop moderately severe or severe psychological problems. Moreover, it should be remembered that the experiencing of an event which threatens loss is strongly correlated with the subsequent onset of psychiatric problems (Brown and Harris 1978).

Anxiety and Depression

To determine the incidence of morbid anxiety and depression in parents, the families of 60 children were followed up during the first 12−18 months after diagnosis of leukaemia at the Royal Manchester Children's Hospital. A group of parents whose children had been admitted and treated for non-life-threatening disease was similarly followed up and acted as a control group. The two groups were closely matched on variables, such as age, marital status, social class and the number of children, that might have influenced the incidence of psychiatric morbidity.
The parents were interviewed within a few weeks of diagnosis and then 12−18 months later by trained interviewers. The interviewers used an abbreviated version of the Present State Examination (Wing et al. 1974) and the Standardised Social Interview (Clare and Cairns 1978) to assess the psychological adjustment of the parents. The parents were also asked to complete the Rutter Behaviour Schedule (Rutter et al. 1970) to assess the incidence of behavioural difficulties in the children.
It was clear from these interviews that most parents reacted initially by finding it very difficult to take in the news that their child had a potentially fatal illness. The onset of leukaemia had usually beeen insidious. The child had complained of symptoms like lack of appetite, tiredness or aches and pains which were easily attributable to minor illness. Even when these persisted, few parents thought that they were due to a serious illness and the news came as a terrible surprise. As the shock set in and parents began to accept that their child was a seriously ill they usually felt very distressed and upset as the following statement by a parent indicates: "When you first learn that your child has such a disease your world collapses. You think: 'it can't happen to us, it only happens to other people!' ". As well as feeling very sad and worried during this postdiagnosis period many parents felt angry and bitter. They questioned why they should have been visited by such an affliction and they

were especially likely to be bitter if they considered that there had been a delay in diagnosis. Yet the doctor may have genuinely mistaken the signs of leukaemia for growing pains, influenza or measles.

These feelings of sadness, anger and worry normally lessen with time and become more manageable. However, the follow-up study showed that in the first few weeks after the announcement of the diagnosis, nearly a third (30%) of mothers were suffering from an anxiety state. They felt on edge, were unable to relax, had great difficulty getting off to sleep because they could not stop thinking about the illness, were experiencing panics occasionally and found that they could not concentrate as well as usual. Only 5% of the mothers of the children who had been admitted for treatment of benign disease were so anxious. There was a similar difference in the incidence of depression. While a third of the mothers of children with leukaemia had developed symptoms of depression including persistent sadness, weepiness, lessening of energy, impaired concentration, impaired appetite and sleep disturbance, only 9% of the mothers of control children had done so. The levels of anxiety and depression at this stage were generally of moderately severe degree and few mothers had become severely depressed. Twelve to 18 months later there was still a substantial difference between the mothers of the leukaemic children compared with the mothers of control children. Fifteen (25%) were suffering from an anxiety state compared with three (5%) of the controls. A similar proportion of the mothers of the sick children (14, 23%) were suffering from a depressive illness at follow-up, compared with four (7%) control mothers. Overall, 17 (28%) of the mothers of leukaemic children were depressed and/or anxious to a morbid degree while only five (8%) of the control mothers were similarly disturbed. Thus, the stress of coping with the child's disease, treatments and attendant hurdles, had caused considerable psychiatric disturbance in a substantial proportion of the mothers.

Similar problems were reported by Peck (1979) and Tiller et al. (1977). The latter authors found that 30% of their mothers had developed a severe or moderate depressive illness, even though they only followed up families where the child had been in remission for some 12–23 months after initial treatment. It seems reasonable to conclude, therefore, that at least one in five mothers will develop morbid anxiety or depression of sufficient severity to warrant help within the first year or so of their child's being diagnosed as having leukaemia. Nor are fathers immune and a substantial proportion may suffer from morbid anxiety or depression (Peck 1979).

It has been suggested (Kaplan et al. 1976) that the incidence of psychiatric problems is greater if the child dies. They followed up 40 families who had lost a child through cancer and found that 11 (35%) of them had at least one member currently in psychiatric care. Even when the child continues in remission for some years up to one in five parents continue to have emotional problems (Duberley 1976).

Sexual Problems of the Parents

In the Manchester follow-up study 20% of those mothers of leukaemic children who had a good sexual adjustment before diagnosis noticed a substantial deterioration in their sexual relationship during follow-up. Eight per cent ceased love-making while 12% got little or no enjoyment from it. Most said that they found it impossible to relax and enjoy lovemaking because they kept thinking about their sick child. They felt guilty that they should enjoy themselves when their child was so ill. Some mothers also said that things had gone wrong sexually because they spent so long in hospital, had become extremely tired and were uninterested in lovemaking when they returned home. A further reason was that some of the affected children were so successful in their insistence that they stay with their parents all the time that they were brought into the marital bed.

Behavioural Problems in the Sick Child

In the Manchester study it was found that 23 (38%) of the 60 children had developed behavioural problems during the follow-up period compared with five (8%) of the control children. The most common problem found was a "dependency syndrome". The parents would describe how the child had become increasingly clinging and dependent and refused to be left alone. When the parents tried to insist that the child spend some time alone, the child would have tantrums, scream and shout. The child was also reluctant to sleep alone. In 12% of children these behavioural problems were severe and caused considerable disruption and unhappiness within the family. The overall incidence of behavioural problems was similar to that found by Howarth (1972) in children suffering from leukaemia (40%) and by Tiller et al. (1977) in children with leukaemia (31%) and other cancers.

Such behavioural problems should be reflected in teachers' observations of these children at school. Eiser (1982) reported that teachers regarded 21% of children with leukaemia as suffering from behavioural problems. They also noted that the leukaemic children were behind with their work compared with their peers and had difficulty maintaining the pace; 22% had required remedial help while 32% were below average in reading and 40% below average in arithmetic. Spinetta and Spinetta (1980) compared 42 children who had been treated for leukaemia or other cancers with 42 healthy children on the basis of teachers' questionnaires. Those treated for cancer had been absent from school more often, were behind in their work, had difficulty with their concentration and learning, were less energetic and less willing to take initiative. Seventeen of them (40%) exhibited behavioural difficulties. Slavin et al. (1982) have suggested that these difficulties persist in 20% of children for several years at least.

Several factors may account for this high incidence of behavioural problems. It may relate to fears about their health and future, and Spinetta and Maloney (1975) have suggested that most children realise what is wrong and become much more preoccupied with their health and bodies than other children. It may also stem from confusion about the nature of their illness when parents have not told the child the truth. The child may then become very perplexed about the way he or she is being treated and find it difficult to reconcile the parents' account of what is wrong with the reality of what is happening. The child might also become disturbed because he or she like the parents is very distressed by the effects of treatment and develops needle phobia or conditioned vomiting. The child may find particular side effects like hair loss especially upsetting since he or she may be the focus of much teasing and even bullying. However well such children try to adapt to these problems, their schooling will be disrupted because of repeated visits to hospital and the advice they are given to stay away from school when there is any risk of their contracting chickenpox or measles.

A further cause for particular concern is the suggestion that treatment causes brain damage and impaired growth (Angio et al. 1978) if given at critical periods of development. It has been claimed that some children show evidence of persistent albeit minor brain damage, are more easily distracted, less able to learn and less able to concentrate than control children. Changes in parents' behaviour also contribute considerably to the development of behavioural difficulties. In the Manchester study over half the parents (55%) found it impossible to continue to treat their child as normal even though advised by the physicians to do so. They became more indulgent, expected much less of the child in terms of self-care and helping around the house, relaxed discipline and expected the child to socialise much less. They reported that the child often took advantage of these changes and became much more difficult to control.

Behavioural Problems In the Siblings

Nearly a third (31%) of the siblings followed up in Manchester developed behavioural problems in the follow-up period although these were usually of less severity than those found in the sick child. This was a lower incidence then that reported by Peck (1979) who found that nearly half of the siblings had experienced problems while Martin et al. (1979) claimed that up to 80% of siblings manifested behaviour or achievement problems. Cairns et al. (1979) gave psychological tests to children with cancer and their siblings. Siblings who perceived their parents as over-protective and over-indulgent of the sick child experienced much greater anxiety, were more worried about their own physical health and felt socially isolated. They also complained of physical symptoms including abdominal pain and headache and said that their own needs were being neglected. Yet they were reluctant to express their worries and anger lest this made matters worse for their parents.
Problems in the siblings who feel left out and neglected are often accompanied by a deterioration in their school performance. Tiller et al. (1977) and Eiser (1983) have reported that changes in behaviour and performance have been noted by teachers in between 20% and 25% of siblings.

Hidden Morbidity

Only one in six of the mothers who developed anxiety, depression or sexual difficulties in the Manchester study had disclosed this to any of the doctors, social workers or nurses concerned in the aftercare of their child with leukaemia. There was, therefore, a serious discrepancy between the needs of these families for help and the care given. Subsequent research has focused on the reasons for this.
The major reason appears to be the reluctance of the parents to take up any of the doctor's time which might otherwise be spent in ensuring that the child receives optimal care. Parents also fear that if they disclose that they are not coping well they will receive little sympathy from the clinicians and other staff who might respond by stressing that it is their duty to cope when their child is so ill. Most parents who had been adversely affected reported that they deliberately put on a brave and false front when they took their child to the hospital for follow-up visits or when they presented to their general practitioner. Since the clinicians and other members of the hospital or community teams focus primarily on the child's physical health many parents remained unconvinced that those responsible for care were concerned about how they were coping psychologically and socially. Even if they were interviewed by social workers or by nurses on the ward or in the community they did not usually disclose how they had been affected.
When asked why they were reluctant to consult their own general practitioner many parents replied that they were sure that the only response they would get would be the prescription of a tranquilliser or sleeping tablet (Comaroff and Maguire 1981). They had

little confidence that the doctor would spend any time identifying and heeding their own real problems.

This claim that doctors did not seem interested in how they were coping might seem unreasonable. However, a detailed study of the doctors who had cared for these children with leukaemia and their parents found that their views were justified. Few general practitioners enquired routinely about how the family was coping and whether there might be any psychological problems. The practitioners gave several reasons for this reluctance to screen for the possibility of problems (Rosser and Maguire 1981). First, they assumed that if families had problems the parents themselves would mention it. Second, if they did enquire about the possibility of problems they might find that they could not deal with them; therefore it was better not to look in the first place. They were particularly concerned that if they enquired too closely about how families were managing they would be asked awkward questions about aetiology and prognosis which they could not answer. They were also worried that they might come face to face with unpleasant aspects of treatment and the reality of what it is like to live with cancer. This might not only upset them but make it difficult for them to function. So, it becomes easier to focus on the physical well-being of the child and avoid any psychological aspects. Some general practitioners gave dramatic accounts of how upsetting it was for them to see a child who had not responded to treatment when they knew that the child had suffered badly from adverse effects of treatment and the parents had questioned the value of it.

Methods of Intervention

Many centres have tackled this problem of adverse psychological sequelae in parents and children by appointing a specialist nurse or social worker. They have done so on the assumption that if such workers provide each family with information, advice, practical help and emotional support from the time of diagnosis onwards they may prevent these difficulties. However, there is still no firm evidence that these assumptions are justified. Indeed, it seems likely that they are not, since it is probably naive to expect that the mere provision of support and advice would do much to buffer the enormous anxiety provoked by knowing that a child has a potentially fatal illness. Moreover, studies of adults with cancer have shown that the provision of support, information and advice does not prevent the incidence of serious problems (Maguire 1982).

In view of the great discrepancy between the families' needs for help and the ability of those involved in their care to recognise these needs it might be better to employ a specialist worker not only to provide help and support but also to systematically monitor their psychological and social progress. If the monitoring were to be effective, the nurse or social worker would need to possess the skills required to enable them to assess whether or not families have developed problems and to know when and to whom they should refer the families for help. While this monitoring approach has proved effective in some adult cancers (Maguire et al. 1980) the impact on families where a child is being treated for leukaemia has yet to be properly evaluated.

Encouraging parents to meet each other in groups to discuss their worries and concerns might also prevent or reduce morbidity. However, there has been considerable concern that groups may be harmful rather then beneficial, particularly if they are dominated by parents who have had adverse experiences of leukaemia and its treatment. On the basis of current evidence it seems likely that, provided these groups are conducted by professionals trained in group methods and fully aware of the predicaments faced by parents as well as being able to control the level at which the group works, they could prove to be of some value (Hefron et al. 1973; Gilder et al. 1978). An alternative is to enlist the aid of volunteers, that is parents who themselves have or have had a child with leukaemia, to advise other parents in the hope that they will feel less isolated and will be more confident that they can cope with the various hurdles. This approach also carries risks unless the parents have had some training in listening and counselling techniques (Steutzer et al. 1976). Moreover, it has to be accepted that some parents prefer not to talk to other parents and they should be given the option of refusing such assistance.

It has been argued frequently that parents are more likely to cope if they take an active role in their child's treatment while the child is in hospital. This may result in one or both parents having too little time out. They may also become too detached from the rest of their family. If families experience profound difficulties a conference with the whole family might prove helpful in identifying and alleviating these (Ablin et al. 1971). Treating the whole family may also be necessary.

Unfortunately, few attempts have been made to evaluate any of these approaches critically in relation to children with leukaemia. Those evaluations that have been conducted have failed to find a substantial effect. For example, Micheletti et al. (1981) assessed a home visit programme where a nurse had been employed to give support to parents and provide any information and help they required. They found little difference between the families helped by the nurse and families who had not received such help. It is worth noting that one of the parents' major criticisms was that the nurse lacked training in counselling techniques and was somehow unable to identify their true needs.

It has also still to be demonstrated that when problems are detected and referred subsequent intervention has a positive impact. Some areas at least appear resistant to change. Fife (1978), in a controlled study, found that it was especially difficult to get parents to go back to treating their child as normal. In some parents, her intervention had the opposite effect to that intended. They became firmer in their view that the child should be over-protected.

The notion of following up all families with a child with leukaemia may be unrealistic. The alternative would be to concentrate only on those families who seem at particular risk of developing difficulties. This will only be viable if it can be demonstrated that certain factors reliably predict the risk of adverse psychological sequelae. Some potential predictors have already been reported. These include: the parents' having an unrealistic view of the child's illness; their being reluctant to discuss the nature of the child's illness openly between themselves and their children; the absence of someone in whom they can confide their true feelings; continuing high levels of distress, anger or guilt; the experiencing of other adverse life events; and the witnessing of serious adverse effects of treatment in the child. Further studies are required to confirm whether these predictors are reliable; if they prove to be so they would provide useful markers of those families most at risk.

Meanwhile, it would seem wise to organise aftercare so that each family is closely monitored during the first months of treatment in such a way that it becomes clear whether the family have developed psychological problems. They can then be offered appropriate help. Careful studies are then needed to see what kinds of intervention make most impact.

References

1. Ablin AR, Binger CM, Stein RC, Kushner JH, Zoger S, Mikkelson C (1971) A conference with
   the family of a leukaemic child. Am J Dis Child 122:362–368

 2. D'Angio GJ, Clatworthy HW, Evans AE, Newton WA, Tefft M (1978) Is the risk of morbidity and rare mortality worth the cure? Cancer 41:377–380
 3. Bodkin CM, Pigott TJ, Mann JR (1982) The financial burden of childhood cancer. Br Med J 284:1542–1544
 4. Brown GW, Harris T (1978) Social origins of depression. Tavistock Publications, London
 5. Cairns NU, Clark GM, Smith SD, Lansky SB (1979) Adaptation of siblings to childhood malignancy. J Pediatr 95:485–487
 6. Clare AW, Cairns VE (1978) Design, development and use of a standardised interview to assess social maladjustment and dysfunction in community studies. Psychol Med 8:589–604
 7. Comaroff J, Maguire P (1981) Ambiguity and the search for meaning: childhood leukaemia in the modern clinical context. Soc Sci Med 158:115–123
 8. Duberly J (1976) The psychological and social impact of childhood leukaemia. MSc thesis, University of Manchester
 9. Eiser CE (1983) How leukaemia affects a child's schooling. Br J Soc Clin Psychol (in press)
10. Fife BL (1978) Reducing parental over-protection of the leukaemic child. Soc Sci Med 12:117–122
11. Gilder R, Buchsman PR, Sitartz AL, Wolff JA (1978) Group therapy with parents of children with leukaemia. Am J Psychother 32:276–287
12. Hefron WA, Bonnelaere K, Master R (1973) Group discussions with the parents of leukaemic children. Pediatrics 52:831–840
13. Howarth RV (1972) The psychiatry of terminal illness in children. Proc Roy Soc Med 65:1039–1040
14. Kaplan DM, Grobstein R, Smith A (1976) Predicting the impact of severe illness in families. Health Soc Work 1:71–82
15. Maguire P (1982) Psychological and social consequences of cancer. In: Whitehouse JM, Tattersall MH (eds) Recent advances in clinical oncology. Churchill Livingstone, Edinburgh
16. Maguire P, Tait A, Brooke M, Thomas C, Sellwood R (1980) The effects of monitoring on the psychiatric morbidity associated with mastectomy. Br Med J 2:1454–1456
17. Martin GW, Goff JR, Powazek M, Payne JS (1979) Psychosocial evaluation of children with cancer. In: Care of the child with cancer. American Cancer Society publication
18. Micheletti R, Patterson RB, Herndon A (1981) Evaluation of a home visitation programme for families of children with cancer. Am J Pediatr/Hematol/Oncol 3:239–245
19. Peck B (1979) Effects of childhood cancer on long-term survivors and their families. Br Med J 1:1327–1329
20. Rosser JE, Maguire P (1982) Dilemmas in general practice; the care of the cancer patient. Soc Sci Med 16:315–322
21. Rutter M, Tizard J, Whitmore K (1970) Education, health and behaviour. Longman, London
22. Slavin LA, O'Malley JE, Koocher GP, Foster DJ (1982) Communication of the cancer diagnosis to paediatric patients: impact on longterm adjustment. Am J Psychiatry 139:179–183
23. Spinetta JJ, Maloney LJ (1975) Death anxiety in the outpatient leukaemic child. Paediatrics 56:1034–1037
24. Spinetta PD, Spinetta JJ (1980) Teachers' appraisal: the child with cancer in school. Am J Pediatr/Hematol/Oncol 2:89–94
25. Stuetzer C, Fuchtman D, Schulman JL (1976) Mothers as volunteers in an oncology clinic. J Pediatr 5:847–848
26. Tiller JWG, Eckhert H, Rickards WS (1977) Family reactions to childhood acute lymphoblastic leukaemia in remission. Aust Paediatr J 13:176–181
27. Wing JK, Cooper JE, Sartorious N (1974) Measurement and classification of psychiatric symptoms. Cambridge University Press, Cambridge

The Childhood Lymphomas

M. G. Mott

Department of Paediatric Oncology, Royal Hospital for Sick Children,
Bristol BS2 8BJ, United Kingdom

Introduction

The leukaemias and lymphomas of childhood account for almost half of the malignant
disease seen in this age group in the Western world. The lymphomas represent 10% of the
total, with an approximately even division between Hodgkin's disease and non-Hodgkin's
lymphoma. Hodgkin's disease was the first of the childhood lymphoid malignancies to
become curable and still has the best prognosis of the group. The prognosis for acute
lymphoid leukaemias improved substantially in the early 1970s but has recently been
overtaken by dramatic advances in the curability of the non-Hodgkin's lymphomas.

Non-Hodgkin's Lymphomas

Unlike Hodgkin's disease, this group of disorders is substantially different from its
counterpart in adults, and there is relatively little overlap between the two age groups.
There is a characteristic form of the disease which presents in the mediastinum, a form
which presents in the abdomen and a mixed group of other forms that present in other
nodal or extranodal sites. Those patients with a mediastinal presentation have almost
exclusively T-cell lymphoblastic lymphoma, a localised form of the disease known as T-cell
leukaemia. Those patients with an abdominal presentation have almost exclusively B-cell
disease. In some of these patients the histological appearance is indistinguishable from the
classic Burkitt's lymphoma that occurs with high frequency in some parts of Africa.
However, the natural history of the disease is quite different, having more in common with
that of the other patients presenting in this country with B-cell disease whose histology is
distinct from that of Burkitt's lymphoma.
Virtually all non-Hodgkin's lymphomas of childhood have diffuse histology, and the
disease should be regarded as systemic at the time of diagnosis in the great majority of
cases. Patients with truly localised disease are uncommon but it is important to distinguish
them, since their treatment should be different. For patients with disseminated disease, the
most urgent priority is to embark on treatment as soon as possible. The number of essential
staging investigations is relatively small. The most important are a bone marrow aspirate
and trephine, and a cytospin preparation of cerebrospinal fluid, because of the propensity
of the disorders in question to spread to the bone marrow and central nervous system.
Patients who do appear to have strictly localised disease need more thourough staging
procedures according to the site of presentation. The most widely used staging system for
non-Hodgkin's lymphomas of childhood is presented in Table 1. It should be noted that
this system takes account of the known natural history of the disease to change the stage.

Recent Results in Cancer Research. Vol. 88
© Springer-Verlag Berlin · Heidelberg 1983

Table 1. Staging system for childhood non-Hodgkin's lymphomas (St. Jude)

Stage I	A single tumour (extranodal) or single anatomic area (nodal), with the exclusion of mediastinum or abdomen
Stage II	A single tumour (extranodal) with regional node involvement Two or more nodal areas on the same side of the diaphragm Two single (extranodal) tumours, with or without regional node involvement, on the same side of the diaphragm A primary gastrointestinal tract tumour, usually in the ileocaecal area, with or without involvement of associated mesenteric nodes only[a]
Stage III	Two single tumours (extranodal) on opposite sides of the diaphragm Two or more nodal areas above and below the diaphragm All the primary intrathoracic tumours (mediastinal, pleural, thymic) All extensive primary intra-abdominal disease[a] All paraspinal or epidural tumours, regardless of other tumour site(s)
Stage IV	Any of the above with initial CNS and/or bone marrow involvement[b]

[a] A distiction is made between apparently localised GI tract lymphoma and more extensive intra-abdominal disease because of their quite different pattern of survival after appropriate therapy. Stage II disease is typically limited to a segment of the gut plus or minus the associated mesenteric nodes only, and the primary tumour can be completely removed grossly by segmental excision. Stage III disease typically exhibits spread to para-aortic and retroperitoneal areas by implants and plaques in mesentery or peritoneum, or by direct infiltration of structures adjacent to the primary tumour. Ascites may be present, and complete resection of all gross tumour is not possible

[b] If bone marrow involvement is present initially, the number of abnormal cells must be 25% or less in an *otherwise* normal marrow aspirate with a normal peripheral blood picture

This is best exemplified by a brief description of the two major forms of childhood non-Hodgkin's lymphoma.

Mediastinal, T-Cell Disease

Most patients who present with a mediastinal mass are adolescent boys. Extensive studies have shown that the malignant clone of cells is derived from T-cells that are often E-rosette positive and acid phosphatase positive. A large panel of monoclonal antibodies which are now freely available indicate that the degree of differentiation of these T cells varies somewhat in those patients who have disease strictly localised to the mediastinum compared to those who present with spread already to the bone marrow, peripheral blood and central nervous system. The natural history of this tumour known as Sternberg sarcoma, is for almost universal spread to bone marrow and meninges to occur unless active steps are taken to prevent this. For this reason all patients presenting with a mediastinal primary are automatically designated as having disseminated disease and are said to be stage III or stage IV, depending on whether or not the bone marrow and central nervous system are found to be involved at the time of diagnosis.

Abdominal, B-Cell Disease

The majority of patients with B-cell disease present with extensive disease throughout the abdominal cavity and frequently with evidence of spread elsewhere; so they too are therefore automatically characterised as having stage III or stage IV disease. A significant subgroup of patients, however, have disease that is apparently localised, usually to the region of the ileocaecal junction, with or without involvement of the regional lymph nodes. These patients may, for example present, with symptoms of intestinal obstruction and at laparotomy the surgeon may be able to resect all macroscopic disease. Before the advent of effective regimes of cytotoxic chemotherapy these were essentially the only patients with abdominal primaries who survived. Their treatment involved radical surgical removal followed by irradiation of the whole abdomen with or without additional chemo-therapy.

Treatment

The treatment for this group of disorders was revolutionised in 1976, when Wollner and her colleagues reported the effectiveness of combination chemotherapy in their primary management, with adjuvant radiotherapy and surgery according to the individual needs of each patient. Our experience using a similar approach for 36 patients who have presented since 1975 is shown in Fig. 1. The actuarial survival and disease-free survival curves indicate that approximately two-thirds of these patients may be expected to have long term control of their disease.

Most of these patients were treated according to the protocol of a national study organised by the United Kingdom Children's Cancer Study Group (UKCCSG). The details of this are

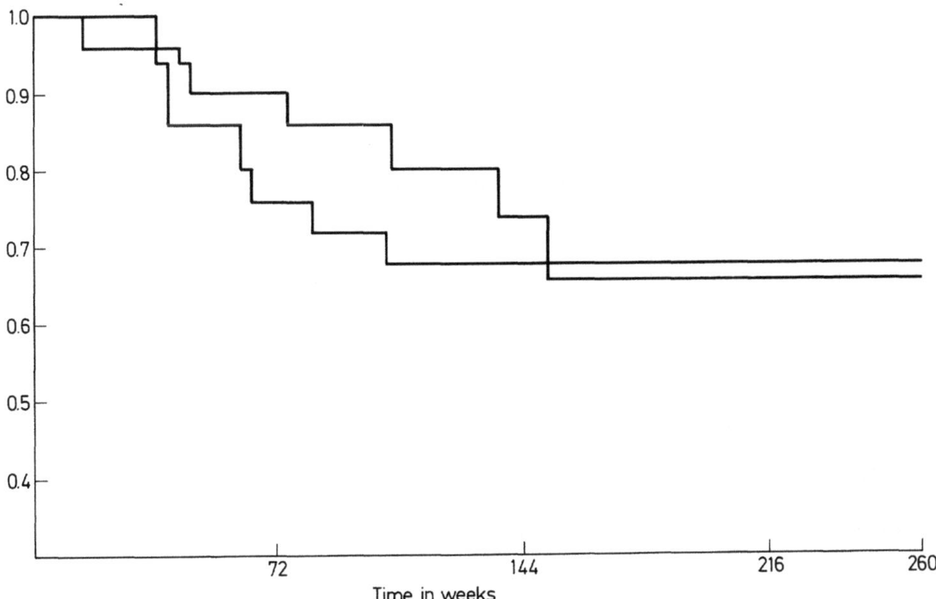

Fig. 1. Actuarial survival and disease-free survival rates of 36 patients with non-Hodgkin's lymphoma treated in Bristol between 1975–1982

Table 2. UKCCSG protocol design for therapy of non-Hodgkin's lymphoma (stages II, III, and IV): intensive combination chemotherapy, with or without radiation to areas of bulk disease

---

Induction

1) CHOP

Cyclophosphamide	1 g/m^2	
Adriamycin	50 mg/m^2	Day 1
Vincristine	1.5 mg/m^2	
Prednisolone	100 mg/m^2	Days 1–5

Given every 3 weeks for 2 cycles

2) Cyt/TG

Cytosine arabinoside	100 mg/m^2 intravenously or subcutaneously 12-hourly for 8 doses
Thioguanine	75 mg/m^2 by mouth daily for 4 doses

Given every 3 weeks for 2 cycles

3) Intrathecal methotrexate   10 mg/m^2 (maximum 12 mg) on day 1 of each course

Consolidation

1) Methotrexate, 500 mg/m^2 (one-third i.v. push, two-thirds i.v. drip over 6 h)

2) 24 h after the beginning of the infusion, folinic acid, 12 mg/m^2 i.m. or i.v., followed by 3 doses of 6 mg/m^2 over the next 24 h

3) Intrathecal methotrexate 10 mg/m^2 at the start of i.v. methotrexate infusion

Given every 2 weeks for 3 cycles

Randomisation

With or without 1,500 rad of radiotherapy to areas of bulk disease, concurrently with consolidation chemotherapy.

N.B. Special category for patients with Sternberg sarcoma

1) Methotrexate 15 mg/m^2 by mouth daily ×4, every 2 weeks for 6 weeks, instead of i.v. methotrexate

2) Intrathecal methotrexate on day 1 of each course

3) Cranial irradiation, 1,760 rad in 8 fractions of 220 rad over 2 weeks

Maintenance

1) Cyclophosphamide/CCNU: Cyclophosphamide 750 mg/m^2 i.v.
                           CCNU 75 mg/m^2 by mouth

2) VM 26 100 mg/m^2 i.v.
Methotrexate 500 mg/m^2 i.v. with citrovorum factor rescue (as in consolidation)
N.B. For patients with Sternberg sarcomas who have received cranial irradiation methotrexate will not be given i.v. but orally at a dose of 12.5 mg/m^2 daily for 4 days.

3) CHOP

Cyclophosphamide	750 mg/m^2
Adriamycin	40 mg/m^2

4) Cyt/TG

Cytosine arabinoside	150 mg/m^2 i.v. or subcutaneously
Thioguanine	75 mg/m^2 by mouth

Given at 3-week intervals. Twelve-week maintenance cycle for 2 years

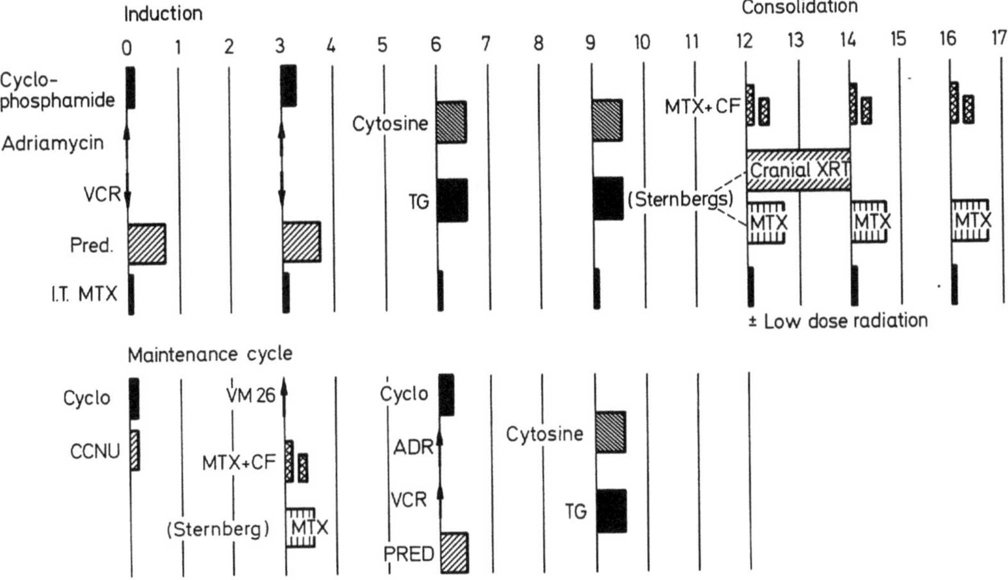

Fig. 2. Summary of the UKCCSG protocol design for treatment of children with non-Hodgkin's lymphoma (stages II, III and IV)

outlined in Table 2 and Fig. 2. The results so far have revealed no additional benefit to the patients randomised to receive radiotherapy in addition to chemotherapy. Analysis of the results for the different subgroups of patients as greater numbers become available should allow improved treatment to be defined for patients with T-cell disease compared to those with B-cell disease.

Hodgkin's Disease

Hodgkin's disease in children appears to be similar in all respects to the disease seen in young adults. It involves a relatively indolent process and spread usually occurs by involvement of contiguous groups of lymph nodes. Current forms of treatment are highly successful and their rationale is perhaps best understood by briefly reviewing the history of their development.

Radiotherapy has traditionally been the standard management for Hodgkin's disease and has effected the cure of many patients with more localised presentations of disease. In children this usually involves painless enlargment of the cervical lymph nodes, unresponsive to antibiotics. The introduction of lymphangiography quickly demonstrated why so many patients relapsed after regional radiotherapy for disease apparently localised above the diaphragm. Relapse would occur in lymph nodes below the diaphragm, since these are not infrequently involved at initial presentation but this was not detected before lymphangiography. The need to confirm equivocal lymphangiogram results by laparotomy and biopsy coupled with the finding of a substantial proportion of patients with occult disease in the spleen led to an era when it was widely regarded as imperative to perform staging laparotomy and splenectomy in all patients. There is no doubt that the

Table 3. UKCCSG, Hodgkin's disease study

Therapy

Stage IA disease − nodal − Involved field radiotherapy
                                    3,500 cGy in 20 fractions in 4 weeks

All other stages (except those with large mediastinal mass)

Chemotherapy − CLVPP	
Chlorambucil	6 mg/m^2 orally for 14 days
Vinblastine	6 mg/m^2 i.v. on days 1 and 8
Procarbazine	100 mg/m^2 orally for 14 days
Prednisolone	40 mg/m^2 orally for 14 days

28-day intervals between 1st day of each course

Treatment should consist of the number of courses taken to achieve clinical remission plus 4 further courses with a minimum of 6 or a maximum of 8 courses.

Non-responders by the end of 3 courses or where there is evidence of progressive disease, change to alternative chemotherapy

---

increased accuracy of staging the disease led to substantially better treatment and a marked increase in the success rate of radiotherapy.

The dramatic regression of far advanced stage III B and stage IV Hodgkin's disease using "MOPP" combination chemotherapy (mustine, oncovin, prednisone, procarbazine) led to further substantial improvements in the treatment of childhood Hodgkin's disease. Two major problems have become apparent: first, the dose of radiation required to cure Hodgkin's disease may have unacceptable effects on growth and development of normal tissues in treated children; secondly, sudden, overwhelming and frequently fatal sepsis may occur in children who have had a splenectomy. Awareness of these problems has led many centres to attempt combined treatment, with low dose radiation to clinically involved lymph nodes and MOPP chemotherapy; this obviated the need for staging laparotomy and splenectomy in all patients, and many of these centres have reported 90% success rates in recent years.

The euphoria induced by these excellent results must however be tempered by consideration of other potential long term complications. There is particular concern about the alarming frequency of reports of second neoplasms, particularly acute myeloid leukaemia (AML) in patients who have received both radiation and chemotherapy for Hodgkin's disease. In view of the extensive projected life span for children cured of Hodgkin's disease this must be a major concern for the future. A less important but nevertheless relevant complication is the possible subsequent sterility of patients who have received MOPP chemotherapy. There is therefore currently a move back towards a policy of treating children with Hodgkin's disease selectively, either with radiotherapy alone or chemotherapy alone. The current UKCCSG treatment study advocates radiotherapy for patients with clinically localised disease (without staging laparotomy and splenectomy), whilst other patients are treated with chemotherapy alone with a less toxic variant of the MOPP programme (Table 3). It is hoped that patients who do relapse following radiotherapy can be successfully managed by subsequent chemotherapy; but it is hoped that most patients will respond adequately to either radiation therapy or chemotherapy alone and so will have reduced risk of developing second malignant neoplasms.

References

1. Dady PJ, McElwain TJ, Austin DE, Barrett A, Peckham MJ (1982) Five years' experience with chlVPP: effective low-toxicity combination chemotherapy for Hodgkin's disease. Br J Cancer 45: 851–859
2. Donaldson SS, Kaplan HS (1982) Complications of treatment of Hodgkin's disease in children. Cancer Treat Rep 66: 977–989
3. Jenkin D, Chan H, Freedman M, Greenberg M, Gribbin M, McClure P, Saunders F, Sonley M (1982) Hodgkin's disease in children: treatment results with MOPP and low-dose extended-field irradiation. Cancer Treat Rep 66: 949–959
4. Mott MG (1980) Chemotherapy of childhood non-Hodgkin's lymphoma. In: Graham-Pole J (ed) Non-Hodgkin's lymphomas in children. Masson, New York, pp 81–94
5. Mott MG (1981) Combination chemotherapy of childhood non-Hodgkin's lymphomas. Cancer Treat Rep (Suppl 1) 65: 119–123
6. Wollner N, Burchenal JH, Lieberman PH (1976) Non-Hodgkin's lymphoma in children. A comparative study of two modalities of therapy. Cancer 37: 123–134

Brain Tumours in Childhood

C. C. Bailey

Regional Department of Paediatric Oncology, Seacroft Hospital,
York Road, Leeds LS14 6UH, United Kingdom

Introduction

Brain tumours are the commonest non-haemopoietic malignancy of childhood. They account for approximately 20% of all newly diagnosed cases of childhood malignancy each year, or approximately 250 new cases per year in the United Kingdom.

In 1980 Ertel published data showing the histological classification of childhood brain tumours diagnosed in the United States between 1973 and 1976. There were 361 cases of which 27% were low grade astrocytoma, 23% were glioma, 22% were medulloblastoma, 10% malignant astrocytoma and 10% ependymoma. Similar data were published from the Connecticut Tumour Registry (Farwell et al. 1977). The data on brain tumours in the Manchester Children's Tumour Registry have been reviewed and reported (Bailey 1979). In the years 1962 to 1976, 323 cases were registered excluding children with oligodendroglioma, optic glioma and craniopharyngioma. Of these cases, 189 (58.5%) were situated in the infratentorial region; 55 of these were benign astrocytomas and 90 were medulloblastomas. Sixty-seven tumours (20.7%) were located in the mid-brain. This location makes surgery extremely hazardous and therefore definitive histological findings were not available on many of the cases. Post mortem studies however indicate that many of them were low grade astrocytomas with occasional medulloblastomas or ependymomas. Fifty-five of the tumours were situated above the tentorium cerebelli; 33 of these were malignant astrocytomas and 13 were ependymomas.

The aetiology of childhood brain tumour remains unknown. The medulloblastoma occurs with decreasing frequency as age increases. This fact and the histological appearance of the tumour cells has led to the hypothesis that the tumour is derived from an embryonic cell line. In contrast the astrocytoma occurs with increasing frequency as age increases and is more likely to be of the malignant, supratentorial type the older the child is at presentation.

Von Recklinghausen's disease (neurofibromatosis) is known to predispose to the development of malignancy and to brain tumour in particular. The Late Effects Study Group of the International Society for Paediatric Oncology (SIOP), is a collaborative group of 12 major North American and European institutions. They have reported at their eighth International Meeting in September 1981 data from two studies which they have undertaken (Bader et al. 1981). In their first study they identified 4968 children with malignancy registered since January 1975, and found amongst them 48 cases of neurofibromatosis compared with an expected incidence of 1.6 cases. Their second study identified 156 families known to have neurofibromatosis and found that for neural tumours the ratio of observed to expected cases was 73.3 in males and 92.9 in females.

Recent Results in Cancer Research. Vol. 88
© Springer-Verlag Berlin · Heidelberg 1983

Surgery and Radiotherapy

The first management which most patients receive for their brain tumour is surgery. The objectives of surgery are threefold. The first, and most important, is to reduce intracranial pressure, by either restoring CSF pathways or by the insertion of a shunt. Secondly, the bulk of tumour must be reduced. Recent results from Philadelphia (Norris et al. 1980) and from the preliminary analysis of an SIOP study, suggest that those patients from whom the neurosurgeon is able to remove the bulk of the tumour have a better prognosis than those from whom only a small amount is removed. The increasing use of the dissecting microscope should enable more extensive and less damaging surgery to be carried out. The third objective of surgery is to obtain adequate tissue for histological examination so that an accurate diagnosis may be made and our understanding of the biology of these tumours *and* their response to different treatment modalities may be improved.

Surgery alone can be an effective cure for the benign cerebellar astrocytoma of childhood in a high percentage of cases. A review of the MCTR data revealed that there were two distinct forms of management for this tumour, surgery alone and surgery followed by radiotherapy to the posterior fossa. Both groups of children showed a 70% ten-year survival rate. It is probable that the children who received radiotherapy were those in whom the neurosurgeon felt that surgery was incomplete. The fact that these children did as well as those not receiving radiotherapy might indicate an advantage in giving radiotherapy to children with residual tumour. This hypothesis needs to be tested by a prospective randomised clinical trial if further light is to be cast upon the subject.

Surgery alone is never curative for medulloblastoma. It is rarely curative for malignant astrocytoma and cannot be utilised for tumours of the midbrain. In all of these situations therefore, radiotherapy plays an important role in increasing the cure rates.

Medulloblastoma sheds cells into the CSF and spinal and cerebral metastases are well described. Radiotherapy must therefore be given to the whole CSF pathway. The Manchester technique is to give 4,500 cGy to the posterior fossa in daily fractions over 6 weeks and 3,000 cGy to the rest of the brain and spinal cord over 4 weeks. A retrospective analysis of the patients treated with this technique at the Christie Hospital and the Holt Radium Institute, Manchester showed a 40% ten-year survival rate. This was comparable to the results from most other major series of patients treated at that time. More recent results obtained from the "no chemotherapy" arms of the SIOP and American Children's Cancer Study Group trials have however shown a considerable improvement on this figure. These increased survival rates may be explained by improved surgical techniques, better post-operative care and possibly more precise radiotherapy techniques. Midbrain tumours are often accompanied by severe neurological deficits and dramatic improvements can sometimes be seen following radiotherapy. The Manchester technique for radiotherapy of these lesions is the same as for medulloblastoma, although the use of the fields to the spine and the cerebrum is debatable. The survival rate is however poor, being only 25%−30% at 5 years.

The malignant astrocytoma infiltrates brain tissue widely and the radiation treatment volume must therefore include the tumour-bearing area with a generous surrounding margin. In practice this usually means irradiating the whole brain. The survival rate is however very poor. None of the tumours situated above the tentorium were associated with survival in the Manchester series although survival rates of up to 30% have been reported from elsewhere (Bloom 1975).

Ependymoma like medulloblastoma may shed cells into the CSF and it has therefore been the Manchester practice to treat it using the same technique as for medulloblastoma. The overall survival rate is 40%–50% at 10 years. Ependymomas vary in their degree of malignancy and whilst all should be regarded as malignant those tumours appearing more "benign" on histological examination could perhaps be treated with a more local radiotherapy field.

Chemotherapy

The results of treatment with surgery and radiotherapy cannot be regarded as satisfactory and in an attempt to improve survival rates the use of chemotherapy has been explored. However, the chemotherapy of brain tumours is complicated by several factors. The principal difficulty is that of delivery of the chemotherapeutic agents to the tumour. It can be shown by infusion studies that in the centre of a brain tumour the normal blood-brain barrier no longer exists; at the interface between tumour margins and normal brain it is commonly intact. The most active and therefore most vulnerable cells of the tumour are unfortunately most likely to be found at the tumour-brain interface. Agents which cannot cross the blood-brain barrier are therefore unlikely to be effective against these tumour cells.

The second problem is that the cell cycle time of most brain tumours is very long and therefore the number of cells entering mitosis during the period of exposure to chemotherapeutic agents is small. Cell cycle dependent agents are therefore unlikely to be of benefit in treating these tumours.

The cytotoxic agent most likely to succeed in the treatment of brain tumours would therefore be a lipid-soluble, non-ionised compound of low molecular weight, i.e. able to cross the blood-brain barrier, and would not be dependent on the cell cycle. Very few drugs fill this description, but the nitrosourea group of compounds were specifically synthethised with these characteristics in mind. Bischlorethyl nitrosourea (BCNU) and cyclohexyl chloroethyl nitrosourea (CCNU) are hydrolysed by the liver to low molecular weight, fat-soluble metabolites which cross the blood-brain barrier and act as alkylating agents. In single agent studies BCNU is slightly more effective than CCNU but has the disadvantage of having to be given as a painful intravenous injection; moreover, BCNU is now well known to cause severe pulmonary fibrosis in some patients (Bailey et al. 1978). Methyl CCNU is less effective against brain tumours than the other nitrosoureas.

Procarbazine is a drug derived from the monoamine oxidase inhibitors. It is metabolised to a fat-soluble azo-compound which crosses the blood-brain barrier and acts as an alkylating agent. Procarbazine has been shown to produce remissions in recurrent tumours of the central nervous system (Edwards et al. 1980).

Vincristine was one of the first drugs to be used in treating brain tumours. Interestingly, it does not cross the blood-brain barrier and it is cell cycle dependent. There is little doubt, however, that it is effective in producing responses in brain tumours, particularly in the early phases of treatment.

Epipodophyllotoxin, VM 26, has also been used in the treatment of brain tumours. It too is fat-soluble but is cell cycle dependent. Response rates of up to 30% in recurrent tumour have been reported (Sklansky et al. 1974). More recently, Sullivan (1979) reporting on behalf of the South West Oncology Group considered that no effect had been demonstrated against childhood brain tumour in their study.

Methotrexate has been extensively studied as a chemotherapeutic agent for brain tumours. Its physical characteristics as a heavily ionised, poorly fat-soluble compound which is cell cycle dependent would argue against its usefulness in this role. However, it can be administered intrathecally and in very high doses intravenously, with folinic acid rescue, which has opened up new possibilities. Reports from Rosen et al. (1977) and Djerassi et al. (1977) suggest that useful responses can be obtained in this way.

National and international trials are now being undertaken of multiple agent chemotherapy used in an adjuvant fashion in the treatment of brain tumours. The SIOP has carried out a trial which has completed recruitment of patients. All patients were managed primarily by surgery and radiotherapy, and were then randomised to receive either no further therapy or adjuvant chemotherapy utilising CCNU and vincristine. Preliminary results suggest that certain of the patients may have benefited from being given chemotherapy.

The American CCSG trial was very similar to the SIOP trial in its design but prednisolone was added to the CCNU vincristine regime. Those patients who relapsed would then receive either procarbazine alone if they had already been given chemotherapy, or vincristine, CCNU and procarbazine if they had been in the control group. This trial is now also closed to patient entry.

Preliminary results are similar to the SIOP findings.

The United Kingdom Children's Cancer Study Group (UKCCSG) is conducting a trial in which patients are randomised to receive either no ongoing chemotherapy or adjuvant treatment with CCNU and procarbazine. This trial is still in progress and results are not yet available.

All three of these trials include a group of patients who do not receive adjuvant chemotherapy. A notable feature of the preliminary analyses is that this "control" group appears to be achieving about a 15%–20% improvement in disease-free survival compared to previously reported series. This may reflect the advantage to patients of inclusion in a controlled trial with the consequent concentration of attention on them and the parallel improvement in treatment techniques. Similar improvements were seen some years ago when children with Wilms' tumour included in the Medical Research Council trial were compared with similar children not included in the trial. These observations also underline once more the inhereant danger of constructing a trial which relies for the interpretation of its result on comparison with "historical" controls.

It is possible that the chemotherapy in these three trials is being administered at a suboptimal time. In the period immediately following surgery the blood-brain barrier is mechanically disrupted and neovascularisation of the tumour is maximal. Delivery of a chemotherapeutic agent at this time should therefore allow it to penetrate the tumour most effectively.

Preliminary studies using this technique were reported to the 1981 SIOP meeting by the West German Cooperative Group (Neidhardt et al. 1981) and by the Amsterdam Group (Voute et al. 1981). The West German Group utilised vincristine, procarbazine and moderate dose methotrexate. The start of radiotherapy was delayed until week 12 after surgery. The Amsterdam Group utilised vincristine and high dose methotrexate, radiotherapy being delayed until week 4 after surgery. Both studies showed that the chemotherapy was well tolerated, did not compromise radiotherapy and that there was no immediate disadvantage to patients in delaying radiotherapy. At the time of the report 28 of 33 patients in the West German study and all 13 patients in the Amsterdam study remained in complete remission. On the basis of these studies a new European study is being designed jointly by the SIOP and the UKCCSG to evaluate the effectiveness of pre-radiotherapy chemotherapy.

References

1. Bader JL (1981) Increased risk of cancer with neurofibromatosis. Abstracts of the XIIIth meeting of the International Society of Paediatric Oncology, p 60
2. Bailey CC (1979) The management of brain tumour in children. In: Morris-Jones PH (ed) Topics in paediatrics. 1. Haematology and oncology. Royal College of Physicians, London, pp 75–83
3. Bailey CC, Marsden HB, Jones PH (1978) Pulmonary fibrosis following therapy with BCNU. Cancer 42: 74–76
4. Bloom HJG (1975) Combined modality therapy for intracranial tumours. Cancer 35: 111–120
5. Djerassi I, Kim JS, Shulman K (1977) High dose methotrexate, citrovorum factor rescue in the management of brain tumours. Cancer Treat Rep 64: 691–694
6. Edwards MS, Levin VA, Wilson CB (1980) Brain tumour chemotherapy: an evaluation of agents in current use for phase II and III trials. Cancer Treat Rep 64 (12): 1179–1205
7. Ertel IJ (1980) Brain tumours in children. CA 30: 306–321
8. Farwell JR, Dohrmann GJ, Flannery JT (1977) Central nervous system tumours in children. Cancer 40: 3123–3132
9. Neidhardt MK (1981) Treatment of medulloblastoma with postoperative chemotherapy before neuroaxis irradiation: an interim progress report on the Berlin pilot study and the West German cooperative trial. Abstracts of the XIIIthe meeting of the International Society of Paediatric Oncology, Marseilles, p 39
10. Norris D, Bruce D, Byrd R, Schut L, Littman P, Bilaniuk L, Zimmerman R, Copp R, Rorke L (1980) Medulloblastoma: improved relapse free survival time with modern management. ASCO Abstracts C287: 21–391
11. Rosen G, Ghavimi F, Niremberg A (1977) High dose methotrexate with rescue in central nervous system tumours in children. Cancer Treat Rep 61: 681–690
12. Sklansky BD, Mann-Kaplan RS, Reynolds AF Jr (1974) 4-Dimethyl-epipodophyllotoxin-B-D-thenylidene glucoside (DTG) in the treatment of malignant intracranial neoplasms. Cancer 33: 460–467
13. Sullivan MP (1979) Non-responsiveness of brain tumours to VM 26 therapy in children. Cancer Treat Rep 63: 155
14. Voute PA (1981) Medulloblastoma: chemotherapy with vincristine, methotrexate and prednisolone in a "sandwich" scheme. Abstracts of the XIIIthe meeting of the International Society of Paediatric Oncology, Marseilles, p 40

Neuroblastoma:
Recent Developments in Assessment and Management

J. Pritchard[1] and J. Kemshead[2]*

[1] Department of Haematology and Oncology, Hospital for Sick Children Institute of Child Health, 30 Guilford Street, London WC1N 1EH, United Kingdom
[2] Imperial Cancer Research Fund Paediatric Oncology Laboratory, Institute of Child Health, London WC1N 1EH, United Kingdom

Introduction

Not all children with neuroblastoma succumb to the disease. "Good-prognosis", "intermediate-prognosis" and "bad-prognosis" patients can now be defined; unfortunately, the latter predominate and give the tumour its overall unsavoury reputation. Children with good-prognosis disease are often cured by surgery alone; by contrast there is little evidence to date of a fall in mortality for bad-prognosis patients. However, neuroblastoma is a chemoresponsive and radioresponsive tumour, and the "tail" on the survival curves published for several series of children treated with combination drug therapy indicate that, even for patients with advanced disease, cure is a less than remote possibility.

Prognostic Features

Staging

The United States Children's Cancer Study Group staging system (the Evans system [Evans et al. 1971]) is commonly used. Despite the biologically arbitrary definition of stage II and stage III disease, depending upon whether or not the tumour crosses the mid-line, discrimination between good-prognosis (stages I and II) and bad-prognosis tumours is achieved. Stage II patients without local lymph node involvement fare better than those with involved nodes. Subclassification of stage II patients into those with (IIA) and without lymph node involvement (IIB) therefore seems sensible (Ninane et al. 1982). That the Evans system is essentially a *surgical* staging method is a disadvantage since surgery is frequently delayed in patients with neuroblastoma. Efforts are under way to introduce the 'TNM' (tumour-node-metastasis) staging system, the precision of which is offset by its apparent complexity.

The delineation of "stage IVs" disease was an important advance in our understanding of the natural history of neuroblastoma (Evans et al. 1981). Such children have a small primary tumour and metastatic disease confined to liver and/or skin and/or bone marrow. They have a much better prognosis than other stage IV patients (Table 1) with spontaneous

---

* The authors gratefully acknowledge secretarial assistance given by Jean Bridger and Elisabeth Moore. Jon Pritchard was supported by the Leukaemia Research Fund, John Kemshead by the Imperial Cancer Research Fund; both authors also received financial support from the Gillian Fabb Memorial Fund and the Sean Browning Cancer Fund

Table 1. Prognosis for children with neuroblastomas related to staging

	% of all neuroblastomas	% 3-year survival
Good prognosis		
Stage I	5	100
IIA	5	90–100
IVs	5–10	70
Intermediate prognosis		
Stage IIB	5	50
Poor prognosis		
Stage III	15–20	10–40[a]
Stage IV	60	10[b]

[a] Range probably reflects variation in interpretation of definition of Evans' stages II and III
[b] Children < 1 year of age have better survival (± 50%) with chemotherapy

regression of tumour occurring in many cases. A recent suggestion (Knudsen and Meadows 1980) that stage IVs disease is a developmental aberration, rather than a cancer, deserves serious consideration. Although the overall survival rate of these patients is around 70% there have recently been worrying reports of late recrudescence of the disease.

Other Prognostic Features

Other features besides stage have been shown to have prognostic significance (Table 2). Both patient age and primary site seem important when analysed as independent variables, but when either stage and age, or stage and primary site are taken *in conjunction,* the importance of stage predominates. This observation confirms clinical suspicion that, compared with children over one year of age, younger patients more frequently have extra-abdominal primaries or early-stage disease at diagnosis. Patients with stage IVs and IV disease who are under one year of age appear to have a similar overall outlook (Table 1). It should however be emphasised that, whereas the stage IVs patients often require minimal therapy, true stage IV patients had as high a mortality before the introduction of chemotherapy as did older patients. Patients diagnosed at age 6 or older appear to show slower evolution of tumour but have as poor an ultimate prognosis as younger patients.

The site of metastasis may also have prognostic significance. Patients with bony secondaries have the worst prognosis of all although it has been suggested that, where only one bony metastasis can be detected, prognosis may be better than for patients with multiple bone involvement.

Ten percent of children with newly-diagnosed neuroblastoma show no demonstrable increase in excretion of urinary catecholamine metabolites; but these patients fare no differently from patients whose levels of vanillyl mandelic acid (VMA) and homo-vanillic acid (HVA) are elevated. However, Laug et al. (1978) have demonstrated that the median survival of patients with urinary HVA/VMA ratios of less than 1 is shorter than that of patients with the reverse ratio. The ultimate survival of the two groups, however, is similar.

Table 2. Prognostic features in children with neuroblastoma

	Favourable	Unfavourable
Stage	(see Table 1)	
Age	< 1 year	
Site	Thoracic	Abdominal except
	Cervical	pelvic
	Pelvic	
Urinary HVA/VMA	< 1	> 1
Histology	Ganglioneuroblastoma	Neuroblastoma
VIP hypersecretion	Present	Absent
Dancing eye syndrome (opsomyoclonus)	Present	Absent

Controversy continues over the prognostic value of histological "differentiation" in tumours. Although patients with stable or spontaneously regressing non-metastatic and even metastatic ganglioneuroblastoma have certainly been described, they are rarities — 1%–2% of all patients in our experience. Most patients with ganglioneuroblastoma have stage I or II disease; histological maturation may not therefore be of independent prognostic significance in previously untreated patients. Recently, "maturation" of previously undifferentiated tumours has been attributed to the components of a specific treatment regime (Raaf et al. 1982). Such assumptions are ill-judged. In these circumstances, it seems much more likely that, after treatment-induced tumour shrinkage, ganglion cells which were actually present at the outset but camouflaged by overwhelming numbers of more chemoresponsive neuroblasts are more easily detected by the histopathologist.

Patients presenting with severe diarrhoea due to vaso-active intestinal polypeptide (VIP) usually have a good prognosis because the responsible primary tumour is almost always either stage I or II. Histologically, these tumours invariably show a high proportion of ganglion cells, which correlates with immunocytochemical evidence that VIP is a product of mature neural elements but not of neuroblasts. Occasionally, serum VIP levels can be useful as a "tumour marker" in the diagnosis of neural crest tumours (Tiedemann et al. 1981).

Diagnosis

Although histopathological evidence is conventionally considered as the only fully reliable way of making a diagnosis of cancer, most paediatric oncologists would now accept combinations of clincial, radiological, cytological and biochemical features in making a diagnosis of neuroblastoma. Table 3 shows details of the scoring system for diagnosis recently introduced by the European Neuroblastoma Study Group. Children who are under stress because of hospital admission and/or acute illness often have slightly elevated urinary VMA levels. The European Neuroblastoma Study Group criteria allow for this by requiring a two-fold increase of VMA and/or HVA excretion before its acceptance as a positive diagnostic criterion. The value of serum catecholamine levels is currently under study and, as in phaechromocytoma, they may prove to be of diagnostic help in the 10%–15% of patients who are "non-excretors" of VMA/HVA. Radiological appearances,

Table 3. European neuroblastoma study group: scoring system for diagnosis

	Points
Histopathological confirmation	2
VMA and/or HVA > 2× normal level for age	1
Characteristic radiology	1
Tumour cells in bone marrow	1
Two points required for diagnosis	

such as a posterior mediastinal mass or a "drooping flower" appearance of one kidney on IVU with suprarenal calcification, may be typical of neuroblastoma but cannot, in isolation, be considered as proof of the diagnosis.

In bone marrow aspirates, neuroblasts cannot be distinguished from other tumour cells by their standard morphology or histochemical appearances. Staining of tumour cells with fluroescence-tagged monoclonal antibodies appears to be much more specific (Kemshead et al. 1982b).

Staging

Staging investigations for newly diagnosed patients are listed in Table 4. A penetrated chest film may reveal posterior mediastinal extension of an abdominal tumour or lymph node involvement that might be missed in a postero-anterior (PA) projection. Lung parenchymal metastases at diagnosis are so rare that a diagnosis of neuroblastoma should be seriously questioned in their presence. For assessment of primary abdominal or thoraco-abdominal tumour and regional lymph nodes, we prefer ultrasound to computed tomography (CT) scanning. The introduction of new generation CT equipment will, however, mean that many of the disadvantages of older equipment (significant radiation dose, requirement for sedation or even anaesthesia, poor quality images in children because of low amounts of body fat) will be overcome. Even now, combined CT scanning'metrizamide myelography has an important role to play in the delineation of "dumb-bell" tumours. There has as yet been no systematic study of the value of liver scanning (^{99}Tc-sulphur colloid) as compared with abdominal ultrasound for detection of metastatic liver disease in neuroblastoma. Our own experience indicates that, where a skilled ultrasonographer is available, liver scans are unnecessary. By contrast, because false negatives occur with either technique we consider bone scanning and skeletal survey to be complementary in the detection of bone secondaries. Claims that gallium scanning can discriminate between good and bad prognosis tumours have yet to be substantiated.

As in many adult solid tumours, infiltration of bone marrow is detected more frequently by examination of marrow trephine biopsy than by examination of aspirates. The yield of positive results is further increased by sampling multiple sites. Trephine biopsy in infants is technically difficult and should be carried out only by experienced operators. Standard haematological and biochemical studies are mandatory before the start of treatment. An elevated blood level of urea or creatinine, for instance, may indicate bilateral renal tract obstruction and may modify the treatment approach.

Table 4. Investigation of children with neuroblastoma

Staging investigations	
1) Essential:	AP and lateral chest film
	Ultrasound ± IVU (20 min film)
	Bone scan and skeletal survey
	Multiple BM aspirates and trephines
2) Optional:	Liver scan
	Gallium scan
Other investigations	
	FBC
	Urea and electrolytes

Treatment

General Principles

The approach to treatment of good-prognosis patients is very different from that for patients with bad-prognosis disease. That many stage I and stage IIA patients fare well after surgery alone implies, paradoxically in this most notorious form of childhood cancer, either that occult micrometastasis is rare in good-prognosis patients or that spontaneous resolution of residual "micro-disease" occurs after removal of the primary tumour. Patients with good-prognosis disease who relapse most likely represent instances of "understaging" especially when historical series of patients, in whom staging has often been performed in a cursory fashion, are under consideration. More careful initial investigation of patients may, in the future, define prognostic groups more precisely.

In our management of bad-prognosis patients, we continue to use combination chemotherapy and delayed surgical removal of the primary tumour.

In our opinion, radiation has no established place in the current therapy of neuroblastoma, except in the management of certain emergencies, such as optic nerve compression or the palliative treatment of bone pain. In the future, total body irradiation (TBI) may be an important component of "high-dose" ablative therapy regimes.

Good-Prognosis Tumours

There is general agreement that for stage I patients surgery alone is satisfactory; however, a difference of opinion still exists as to the value of postoperative treatment in patients with stage II disease, even without local node involvement (stage IIA). Stage IIA patients are so rare (about five annually in the United Kingdom) that a definitive answer to this question is unlikely to come from prospective randomised studies. Rather, it seems more appropriate to stage good-prognosis patients exhaustively and to follow them carefully, regularly repeating staging investigations even in clinical remission to determine the rates and patterns of recurrence. A provocative observation in stage II patients is that children with "dumb-bell" primary neuroblastomas who have total or subtotal resection of the intraspinal, extradural component of the mass but no further treatment for the gross residual extraspinal disease may survive without further evidence of actively growing

Table 5. Survival of previously untreated bad-prognosis patients after combination chemotherapy

Regimen[a]	2-year disease-free survival (%)	Reference
C, V	22[b]	9
C, V, A	17.5[b]	9
C, V, A	17	10
C, V, DTIC	23	11
C, V, A, DTIC	18	11
C, V, A, HDM	30[b]	12
C, V, PAP, f3TdR	28	13

C, cyclophosphamide; *V*, vincristine; *A*, adriamycin; *DTIC*, dimethyl triazeno imidazole carboxamide; *HDM*, high dose melphalan; *PAP*, papaverine; *f3TdR*, trifluorothymidine
[a] Incidence of surgical removal of primary tumour is unclear for some series
[b] Includes some stage III patients; otherwise stage IV only

tumour. Again, the rarity of patients in this clinical category dictates against prospective controlled studies of the value of postoperative therapy. Our present policy is to advise no postoperative treatment for carefully staged IIA patients.

Babies with stage IVs disease are managed conservatively by most clinicians in the hope that spontaneous resolution of disease will take place (Evans et al. 1981). Low dose radiation or chemotherapy and/or insertion of a silastic patch in the abdominal wall are sometimes life saving when massive hepatomegaly causes respiratory embarrassment. The primary tumour is conventionally resected after resolution of metastatic disease but there is no hard evidence to suggest that this is actually necessary.

Intermediate-Prognosis Disease (Stage IIB)

It is our present policy to give children four courses of postoperative OPEC chemotherapy (oncovin, *cis*-platinum, epipodophyllotoxin-VM26 and cyclophosphamide) in an effort to reduce the rate of metastatic relapse. Patient numbers, at present, are too small to justify comment on the efficacy of this approach.

Bad-Prognosis Tumours

Children with bad-prognosis disease are conventionally treated with combination pulsed chemotherapy with attempted removal of the primary tumour in partial responders. There is little evidence, to date, that the cure rate has improved as a result of this approach (Ninane et al. 1981; Gasparini et al. 1974; Finkelstein et al. 1979; Pritchard et al. 1982; Nitschke et al. 1980) (Table 5). However, a majority of patients (55%–90% depending upon the regime) obtain complete symptomatic relief with chemotherapy and enjoy a good quality of life. In our hands, the proportion of patients achieving "good partial response" (i.e. disappearance of all subjective and objective evidence of metastases and shrinkage of primary tumour by more than 50% in each of three dimensions) has been increased by the addition of *cis*-platinum and VM 26, sequentially timed for maximum cell kill (Hayes et al. 1981).

Patients achieving good partial response have, of course, a significantly longer symptom-free period than do patients with a mixed, partial or no response to chemotherapy (Ninane et al. 1981). The OPEC regime (see above) has recently been adopted for children with bad-prognosis disease (Pritchard et al. 1981). Although high doses of alkylating agents are undoubtedly capable of shrinking tumours resistant to standard doses of chemotherapy (Pritchard et al. 1982), it has yet to be shown that the use of high-dose "consolidation" therapy, for example with melphalan, can have an impact on the natural history of neuroblastoma. Members of the European Group are therefore studying two other questions in these patients:

1. In children who achieve good partial response after OPEC and surgical removal of the primary tumour, does a single course of high-dose melphalan ($180\,mg/m^2$) with autologous bone marrow rescue delay the time to relapse and/or improve ultimate survival?
2. Compared with historical series, does cessation of all chemotherapy after 9−10 months prejudice the duration of disease-free survival in these patients? In other words, is there a role for maintenance therapy in bad-prognosis neuroblastoma?

Future Prospects

In our experience (Ninane et al. 1981; Pritchard et al. 1982), most patients relapsing after chemotherapy do so at metastatic sites. There are three possible explanations for this:

1. Chemotherapy, even in high doses, fails to ablate residual tumour in patients;
2. Occult tumour cell contamination of bone marrow (aspirated and stored prior to delivery of high-dose chemotherapy) reseeds the patient with metastatic disease;
3. Both these mechanisms are operative.

Research effort has, therefore, recently been directed towards the identification of new chemotherapeutic agents and treatment strategies and also towards improving methods for detection of occult tumour cells in bone marrow.

In experimental studies, using the CHP100 human neuroblastoma cell line and a clonogenic assay, the activity of individual drugs has been shown to parallel their clinical activity (Hill and Whelan 1981). The drugs mAMSA, *cis*-platinum, adriamycin and VM 26 were found to be particularly effective in this system, which can also give some information about dose-response relationships. High single-dose therapy using melphalan and/or cyclophosphamide, and in some centres high-dose drug therapy combined with total body irradiation, together with either autologous or allogeneic bone marrow transplantation, can lead to impressive tumour shrinkage. Occasional survivors, even after treatment of relapsed disease, are seen. Perhaps in vitro studies or in vivo work with nude mice bearing xenografted human neuroblastoma may provide guidelines as to how best to combine chemotherapy and total body irradiation so as to maximise the therapeutic ratio in clinical practice.

Several years ago we began to manufacture antibodies which we hoped would differentiate between neuroblasts and bone marrow cells. Such reagents would, it was felt, be of diagnostic and therapeutic use. Because of their precise specificity we chose to make monoclonal reagents rather than hetero-antisera. Fig. 1 is an illustration of the discriminant capacity of these antibodies. They were made principally by immunising BALB-c mice with human foetal brain followed by fusion of these animals' spleen cells to BALB-c murine

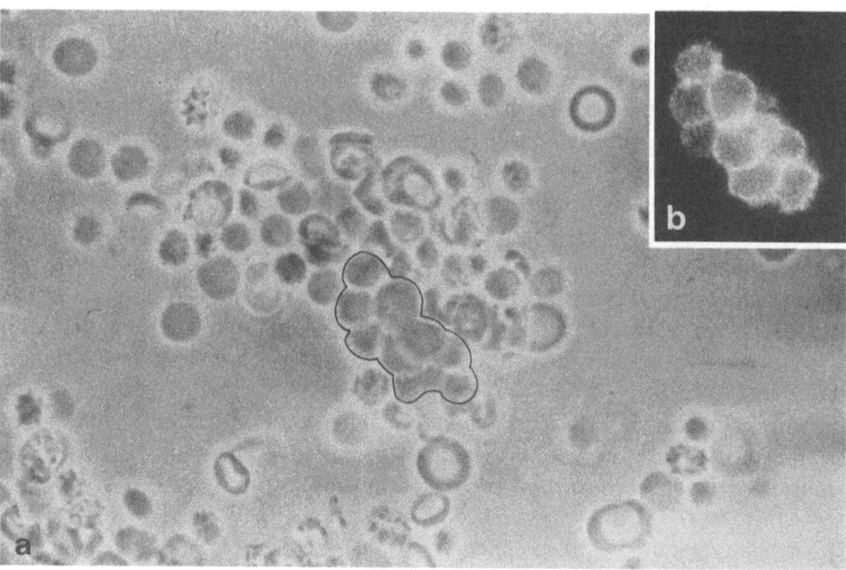

Fig. 1. a Phase contrast photograph of bone marrow suspension from child with newly diagnosed stage IV neuroblastoma; **b** photograph of same microscopic field as in **a** viewed under ultra-violet light. A group of neuroblasts are identified by binding of fluorescence-tagged monoclonal antibody UJ13A. The surrounding normal bone marrow cells do not bind the antibody

myeloma cells. Neuroblasts can now be detected down to, but not below, 0.1% of the nucleated marrow cell population. Recent work has shown that there is considerable heterogeneity of antigen expression within and between individual primary and secondary neuroblastomas, and that, to maximise the chance of tumour cell binding, it is necessary to use a panel of monoclonal reagents. For instance, in a recent study, only 21 of 38 tumours expressed the antigen recognised by all eight of a panel of antineural monoclonal antibodies whilst three expressed only four antigens (in different combinations) and 14 expressed an intermediate number (Kemshead et al. 1982b). Variation of antigen expression has also been identified in different metastases from the same patient at the same point in time and also in sequential studies of the same metastatic site (bone marrow) in the same patient (Malpas et al. 1982). Variability of cell surface antigen expression has been demonstrated in several malignancies. Patterns of antigen expression by neuroblasts may correlate with the various clinical patterns of disease and with histopathological variation, e.g. differentiation, as has been shown in acute lymphoblastic leukaemia (ALL). At least some of the antigens binding these antineural reagents are present in normal tissues. The antibody UJ127.11, for instance, binds to neural but not to glial cells. It is interesting to speculate that naturally occurring antibodies to particular neuroectodermally-associated antigens on neuroblastoma cells may cross-react with other neural tissues and cause specific neurological syndromes such as opsoclonus-myoclonus and cerebellar ataxia.

There are other interesting possible uses for monoclonal reagents. Using nude mice bearing tumours derived from one of our patients, we have recently been able to show efficient selective targeting of UJ13A radio-labelled with ^{123}I to implanted neuroblastomas (Goldman et al. 1983) and we are now starting to apply the same technique to children. Whilst the therapeutic use of antibodies in vivo is not yet a reality, the reagents can be used to remove residual tumour cells from bone marrow before autologous transfusion. Given a maximum detection sensitivity for tumour cells of 0.1% (see above), the standard dose of $2-4 \times 10^9/l$ nucleated marrow cells reinfused in an autologous transplant procedure could harbour $2-4 \times 10^6$ neuroblasts. Various techniques (complement-mediated cell killing, killing by antibody-targeted drugs or toxins, fluorescence-activated cell sorting and differential centrifugation) have been investigated as possible ways of eliminating residual tumour cells. Currently, we favour the use of magnetite-containing polystyrene microspheres coated with antibodies. In laboratory studies of artificial mixtures of neuroblasts and normal marrow cells, efficient separation ($> 99\%$) of the two cell populations is achieved by passing the mixture through a magnetic field (Kemshead et al. 1983).

Conclusions

To paediatric oncologists, neuroblastoma remains the most vexing solid tumour of all. Though almost all good-prognosis children survive disease-free after minimal treatment, the majority of children with advanced disease eventually die of the tumour. More careful staging and more precise definition of prognostic factors will improve our understanding of the disease. The introduction of new chemotherapeutic agents and of better techniques of delivering both cytotoxic drugs and radiation therapy should improve the prognosis for these children. In no other area of childhood malignancy is collaboration between basic laboratory scientists and clinicians more likely to be fruitful.

References

1. Evans AE, D'Angio GJ, Randolph J (1971) A proposed staging for children with neuroblastoma. Cancer 27: 374−378
2. Evans AE, Baum E, Chard R (1981) Do infants with stage IVs neuroblastoma need treatment? Arch Dis Child 56: 271−274
3. Finkelstein JZ, Klemperer M, Evans AE (1979) Multi-agent chemotherapy for children with metastatic neuroblastoma: a report from the Children's Cancer Study Group. Med Pediatr Oncol 6: 179−188
4. Gasparini M, Fossati-Bellani F, Musumeli R, Bonadonna G (1974) Response and survival of patients with metastatic neuroblastoma after combination therapy with adriamycin, cyclophosphamide and vincristine. Cancer Chemother Rep 58: 365−370
5. Goldman AJ, Vivian GC, Gordon I, Pritchard J, Kemshead JT Immunolocalisation of neuroblastoma using radiolabelled monoclonal antibodies. Proc Amer Soc Clin Oncol (Abstr C-271) 19: 70
6. Hayes FA, Green AA, Casper J, Cornet J, Evans WE (1981) Clinical evaluation of sequentially scheduled cisplatin and VM 26 in neuroblastoma. Cancer 48: 1715−1718
7. Hill BT, Whelan RDH (1981) Assessment of the sensitivities of cultured human neuroblastoma cells to anti-tumour drugs. Pediatr Res 15: 1117−1122
8. Kemshead JT, Rembaum A, Ugelstad J (1982a) The potential use of monoclonal antibodies and microspheres containing magnetic compounds to remove neuroblastoma cells from bone marrow to be used in autologous transplantation programmes. Proc Am Soc Cancer Res Proc Am Soc Clin Oncol (Abstr C143) 23: 36
9. Kemshead JT, Goldman A, Fritschy J, Malpas JS, Pritchard J (1983) The use of panels of monoclonal antibodies in the differential diagnosis of neuroblastoma and lymphoblastic malignancy. Lancet 1/8: 12−15

10. Knudson AG, Meadows AT (1980) Regression of neuroblastoma IVs; a genetic hypothesis. N Engl J Med 302: 1254–1256
11. Laug WE, Siegel SE, Shaw KNF, Larsding B, Baptiste J, Gutenstein M (1978) Initial urinary catecholamine metabolite concentrations and prognosis in neuroblastoma. Pediatrics 62: 77–82
12. Malpas JS, Kemshead JT, Pritchard J, Greaves MF (1982) Heterogeneity in cell surface antigens on human neuroblastoma cells. In: Proceedings of the XIIIth meeting of the International Society of Paediatric Oncology. Excerpta Medica, Amsterdam pp 90–94
13. Ninane J, Pritchard J, Malpas JS (1981) Chemotherapy of advanced neuroblastoma: does adriamycin contribute? Arch Dis Child 56: 544–548
14. Ninane J, Pritchard J, Morris-Jones P, Mann JR, Malpas JS (1982) Stage II neuroblastoma: adverse prognostic significance of lymph node involvement. Arch Dis Child 57: 438–442
15. Nitschke R, Cangir A, Crist W, Berry DH (1980) Intensive chemotherapy for metastatic neuroblastoma. Med Pediatr Oncol 8: 281–288
16. Pritchard J, Shafford EA, Craft AE, McElwain TJ (1981) High doses melphalan (HDM) with autologous bone marrow (ABM) for advanced neuroblastoma. Proc Am Soc Clin Oncol (Abstr C 307) 22: 410
17. Pritchard J, McElwain TJ, Graham-Pole J (1982) High dose melphalan with autologous marrow for treatment of advanced neuroblastoma. Br J Cancer 45: 86–98
18. Raaf JH, Cangir A, Luna M (1982) Induction of neuroblastoma maturation by a new chemotherapy protocol. Med Pediatr Oncol 10: 275–282
19. Tiedemann K, Long RG, Pritchard J, Bloom SR (1981) Plasma vaso-active intestinal polypeptide and other regulatory peptides in children with neurogenic tumours. Eur J Pediatr 137: 147–150

Wilms' Tumor

P. H. Morris Jones

Department of Paediatric Oncology, Royal Manchester Children's Hospital,
Manchester M27 1HA, United Kingdom

Introduction

The current results of the treatment of nephroblastoma are one of the success stories of
paediatric oncology. One of the first recorded reports of a nephrectomy for a Wilms'
tumour was by Mr. Jessop at Leeds Infirmary, who in 1877 reported in the Lancet
(Annotations 1877); Max Wilms wrote his monograph on the tumour in 1899. Review of
the literature shows that surgery alone, which was the usual treatment in the first half of this
century, achieved cure rates of approximately 20%. These results were improved by the
addition of radiation therapy, the first recorded case treated being reported by Friedlander
(1916). The apparatus used was a Coolidge tube and the patient concerned had a tumour so
large that no surgeon was willing to undertake its removal. There was a good response to
treatment though this was short lived. The combination of radiotherapy and surgery
improved survival rates significantly and until the 1950s this treatment was standard in most
centres. Properative irradiation was relatively common; there was usually good response
with reduction in the size of the tumour and subsequent removal was facilitated. In the
situation where primary removal was possible it was usually the treatment of choice and
this allowed the surgeon and pathologist to assess the extent of the spread of the
tumour.
Chemotherapy in the treatment of nephroblastoma was not used with any frequency until
Farber et al. (1956) demonstrated efficacy of actinomycin D. Previous reports of the use of
chemotherapy included the use by Coley (1935) of toxins. From the time of Farber's report
chemotherapy has become an increasingly important part of treatment and in some stages
of the disease is now replacing radiotherapy.

Clinical Manifestations

Presentation

Nephroblastoma can present at any age; it has been reported at birth and in the elderly but
the peak incidence is in the second and third years of life and more than 75% of patients
present before the age of 5 years. The ages of 129 children treated in Manchester between
1954 and 1978 are shown in Fig. 1. In larger series a slight male preponderance of about
1.2 : 1 has been found and in the series described here it was 1.1 : 1. There is no significant
difference in the frequency with which the tumour occurs on the right or left. Bilateral cases
account for about 5% of patients in large series; however, bilaterality has been reported in
a higher percentage of patients from some centres, but this is likely to be due to a referral

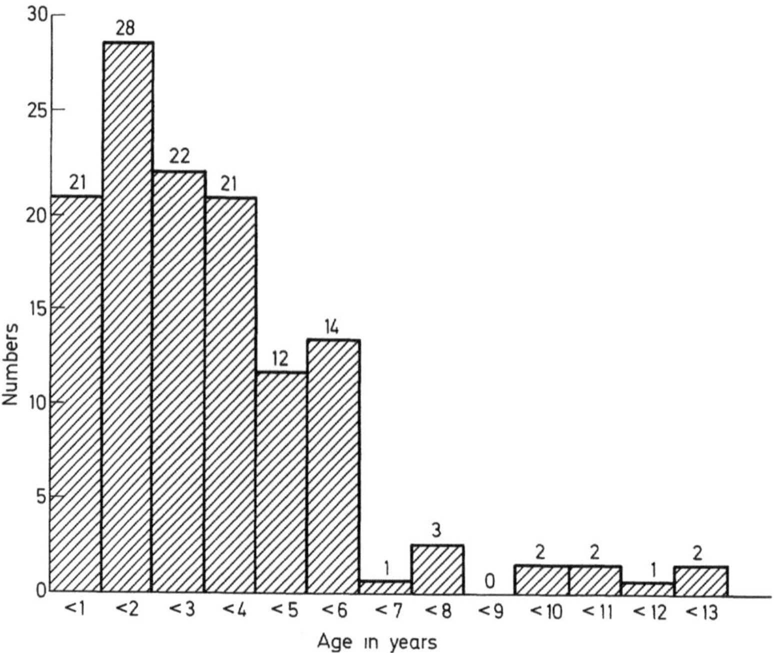

Fig. 1. Ages of 129 children treated for nephroblastoma in Manchester between 1954 and 1978

bias. There were six bilateral cases in the Manchester series and as this is a population-based series it is likely to represent the true frequency.

The commonest mode of presentation of Wilms' tumour is as a palpable abdominal mass which is usually detected by the parents. The child is often otherwise healthy and associated symptoms are rare. Abdominal pain may be a complaint in older patients and overt haematuria is reported in approximately a quarter of patients. On examination it is usual to find a firm non-tender mass in the upper abdomen. The tumour and kidney together tend to retain a reniform shape and it is uncommon for the mass to cross the mid line. Although it is palpable in the loin it is not usually completely fixed and unless there has been gross rupture of the renal capsule it has a smooth outline.

Tumour Markers

A proportion of children with nephroblastoma have hypertension, thought to be associated with increased renin activity. In some cases this seems to be due to autonomous production of renin by the tumour; after falling to normal levels when the primary tumour has been removed, it may rise again with the development of metastatic disease. In other cases excess renin production is probably due to compression of the renal artery by the tumour.

A small proportion of children with nephroblastoma may have polycythaemia secondary to increased erythropoietic activity. A mucopolysaccharide in the serum of a child with nephroblastoma was reported by Morse and Nussbaum (1967) and further reports occurred in the early 1970s. It was suggested at that time that it might be a useful marker in the disease but this has not been followed up.

Associated Abnormalities

Nephroblastoma has been shown to be associated with other congenital abnormalities. There are many cases reported with renal tract abnormalities including duplex systems, horseshoe kidney, hypospadias and pelviureteric obstruction. It is difficult to be sure whether these are random associations as the frequency is not established in the population as a whole. There is however a definite association with hemihypertrophy. This overgrowth of one side of the body, or occasionally of just one limb or one side of the face, is estimated to occur in approximately one in 15,000 births. Its incidence in association with nephroblastoma is between one in 15 and one in 32. Sporadic anirida occurs in one in 50,000 births, while it is found in about one in 50 children with nephroblastoma. These children also frequently have some or all of the following: cataracts, mental retardation, hypospadias and undescended testes. They have all been shown by Ladda et al. (1974) to have a chromosomal abnormality — a deletion of the short arm of chromosome 11. Children with familial aniridia, or sporadic aniridia without Wilms' tumour do not have chromosome anomalies. There is also an increased incidence in association with the Beckwith-Weidemann syndrome. This syndrome, characterised by macroglossia, organomegaly, umbilical hernia or exomphalos, is a rare condition. It has an association with other paediatric malignancies including adrenal carcinomas, gonadal tumours and hepatoblastomas and also benign haematomas. Cases have also been described with associated hemihypertrophy; and associations have been reported with pseudohermaphroditism and progressive renal failure due to glomerulonephritis by Barakat et al. (1974).

Familial Cases

There have been several reports of nephroblastoma occurring in more than one member of the same family. In such patients the frequency of bilateral cases is increased and they also occur on average in a younger age group.

Management

Investigations

The clinical evaluation of the child with an abdominal mass must of course be confirmed by investigations. A full blood count is necessary to exclude anaemia which may be present if there has been haemorrhage into the tumour. Measurement of blood urea and electrolytes will exclude any gross renal dysfunction and a routine examination of the urine will establish whether or not there is haematuria. Mandatory radiological examinations are confined to an IVU and high quality standard x-rays of the chest — both P.A. and lateral films.
Ultrasonography is increasingly used and has the advantage of being non-invasive. In the hands of an experienced radiologist it can be used to establish the patency of the inferior vena cava and whether or not tumour thrombus is present. Nodal enlargement may also be detected and hepatic metastases may be demonstrated if they are of considerable size. It is doubtful however whether any of these findings should actually influence the plan of management at present.

Computerised tomography of the lungs and abdomen may also add some information to the initial findings. It must however be borne in mind that sedation will be necessary to obtain high quality definition in young children. In addition, for proper assessment of the lungs cooperation with breath holding is necessary so that there is a limit to the accuracy of the scans in the determination of lung metastases. The high dose of radiation involved should act as a deterrant to the routine use of scans. It is important to remember that while computerised tomography may detect otherwise occult metastases the majority of children with nephroblastoma are at present being cured by current methods. The intensification of treatment on the basis of the detection of more widespread disease by these newer techniques may not be necessary and may prevent the delineation of those cases in which different therapy may be of use. At present therefore, large centres with a significant throughout of patients should be using the newer techniques to establish as accurately as possible the extent of disease while maintaining current policies of treatment. When sufficient information has been acquired it will be possible to select those patients who have features at diagnosis implying a poor prognosis.

Surgery

In the United Kingdom and North America there is little argument that nephrectomy should be the first line of management in the majority of patients with nephroblastoma. It is only in a minority of children that this is not possible. Preoperative rupture of the tumour is a rare finding and provided a large transabdominal, transperitoneal incision is used, together with careful dissection, intra-operative rupture is also uncommon. There is no evidence that minor spill at operation is of prognostic significance.
The policy in the rest of Europe is to use preoperative chemotherapy or radiotherapy to reduce the size of the tumour and facilitate its complete removal. The survival rates associated with these different methods are comparable and it seems likely that the policy in Europe has evolved because of a tendency for children to present with later stage disease and larger tumours (Lemerle et al. 1976).

Staging

The current management of children with nephroblastoma is highly dependent on accurate surgical and pathological staging. Various systems have been devised but the most commonly used and most widely accepted is that devised by the National Wilms' Tumour Study Group (NWTS) in the United States. It is based on an assessment of the extent of the disease at the time of diagnosis and confirmation of the surgeon's findings by the pathology laboratory. The staging presently advocated has been described by Farewell et al. (1981) and given in Table 1. These stages have been evolved by careful analysis of prognostic factors in large numbers of patients whose tumours have been examined in considerable detail by a panel of pathologists. In many patients, multiple biopsies have been taken from various specified sites; for example, hilar and para-aortic nodes which appear involved are sampled by the surgeons and carefully labelled before being sent for histological examination.
As a result of these detailed analyses pathologists have also been able to describe variants of the classical description of nephroblastoma. In addition to the typical Wilms' tumour three other types, described as anaplastic, rhabdoid and bone metastasising (or clear cell),

Table 1. Stage grouping of Wilm's tumour

Stage I	Tumour limited to the kidney and completely excised. Surface of renal capsule intact. Tumour has not ruptured before or during removal. No residual tumour apparent beyound the margins of resection
Stage II	Tumour extends beyond the kidney but is completely excised. There ist regional extension of the tumour, i.e., penetration through the outer surface of the renal capsule into perirenal soft tissues. Vessels outside the kidney substance are infiltrated or contain tumour thrombus. The tumour may have been biopsied or there may have been local spillage of tumour comfined to the flank. No residual tumour apparent at or beyond the margins of excision
Stage III	Residual non-haematogenous tumour confined to the abdomen. Any one or more of the following may occur: a) Lymph nodes are found on biopsy to be involved in the hilus, the peri-aortic chains or beyond b) There has been diffuse peritoneal contamination by the tumour, e.g. by spillage beyond the flank before or during surgery or by growth of the tumour causing penetration through the peritoneal surface c) Implants are found on the peritoneal surfaces d) Tumour extends, either microscopically or grossly, beyond the surgical margins e) Tumour is not completely resectable because of local infiltration into vital structures
Stage IV	Haematogenous metastases; deposits beyond stage III, i.e., lung, liver, bone and brain
Stage V	Bilateral renal involvement at diagnosis

are now recognised (Beckwith and Palmer 1978; Marsden and Lawler 1978, 1980). These three types make up about 12% of large series of renal tumours in childhood and carry a poor prognosis.

The pathologist must also recognise the mesoblastic nephroma and nodular renal blastema neither of which are malignant pathological entities but may on occasion be associated with nephroblastoma (Bolande 1974; Beckwith 1970, 1974). Once the stage of the tumour has been established and the histologic subtype defined further therapy can be decided upon. As very large numbers of children have now been treated according to well defined protocols and the outcome monitored it is possible to advise treatment programmes which have a very high success rate and which minimise toxicity and side effects.

Chemotherapy

The effectiveness of actinomycin D and vincristine in the treatment of the tumour was established in the 1950s and 1960s. Children have been cured by surgery, radiation therapy and actinomycin D and yet different protocols have produced very different disease-free survival and overall survival rates. This suggests that the actual scheduling of the drugs is very important. It was reported that multiple courses of actinomycin D were more effective than a single course by the study of the Children's Cancer Study Group (C.C.S.G.) in the United States (Wolff et al. 1968). The design of this study carried a bias in favour of multiple courses in that children were not randomised to receive such treatment unless they were disease-free at the time the second course of chemotherapy was due. A subsequent study by the European based International Society of Paediatric Oncology (SIOP) did not show any difference between a single course and multiple courses of actinomycin D (Lemerle et al. 1976). The first study of the Medical Research Council (MRC) (Morris Jones et al. 1978) had 11 patients who relapsed following radiation therapy before the first course of maintenance chemotherapy. These patients proved very resistant to further treatment, suggesting that they formed a particularly bad prognostic group and similar patients might have been important in the bias in the CCSG study.

Vincristine has been used as the only cytotoxic agent in other studies. In the MRC first study all children with stage I disease who were given this regime survived. The drug was given weekly for 10 weeks and then every 2 weeks for 2 years. This was an intensive and prolonged treatment regime, and neurotoxicity was experienced by a proportion of patients. In the second study, as yet unpublished a less intensive regime was used and treatment with Vincristine for year was compared with treatment for 6 months. The survival rates in both arms are in excess of 90% and no advantage is shown for the longer course.

Trials I and II of the NWTS in the United States were designed to answer certain specific questions. The first trial demonstrated that with the protocols used double agent chemotherapy (actinomycin D and vincristine) was superior to either agent alone. This study also indicated that in young patients with stage I tumours radiotherapy was not necessary. This was an important advance, as the long term effects of radiation are significant in this group of children (D'Angio et al. 1976).

The NWTS therefore examined whether by giving double agent chemotherapy to stage I patients irrespective of age they could omit radiatiotherapy without detriment. This was shown to be the case by D'Angio et al. (1979). In view of this the United Kingdom Children's Cancer Study Group (UKCCSG) are now examining the effectiveness of vincristine alone in stage I patients following primary nephrectomy. This study has only been underway for 18 months and results are not yet available. The NWTS, MRC, UKCCSG and SIOP have all examined the use of adriamycin in patients with more extensive disease. The American group have shown an advantage while the other groups have not.

Radiotherapy

Radiotherapy should now be given as a routine only to patients with stage II, III, and IV disease. The volume treated should include the renal bed with 2-cm margins superiorly, inferiorly and laterally and 2 cm beyond the mid line medially so that the whole width of the vertebral bodies is included. Parallel opposed fields should be used and the dose should be 2,000 cGy in 180 cGy or 200 cGy fractions 5 times weekly until the total dose is achieved. Treatment would therefore normally be completed in 15 or 16 elapsed days. Both fields should be treated each day.

In stage III and IV cases where the surgeon finds disease outside the limits described above, the field should be extended in continuity to include all involved areas. If in these circumstances the remaining kidney is included in the field it should be shielded from the posterior field throughout.

In individual cases other fields and techniques may be appropriate. These children should be treated in large centres with considerable experience of the complications of therapy.

If pulmonary irradiation is to be given both lungs should be treated including the apices and postero-inferior portions regardless of the number or location of metastases. The dose advised is 1,200 cGy in 8−10 daily fractions.

Special Problems

One of the most important facts to have emerged from these studies has been the poor prognosis associated with the rare histological variants previously described. While these variants account for approximately 10%−12% of all the cases in the studies they account for more than 50% of the fatal cases.

The present methods of treatment are clearly highly successful for children with the classical histological appearance of nephroblastoma; but these methods are not achieving acceptable results in the subgroups mentioned above and likewise in children who have stage IV disease at diagnosis. Current studies are therefore looking at the following new approaches: the inclusion of other drugs in the chemotherapeutic regimes, the effectiveness of "second look" laparotomies after chemotherapy in children with inoperable primaries and unfavourable histology, and late irradiation. At the same time every effort is being made to define prognostic factors and to refine therapy so that children receive no more treatment than is necessary to ensure success. Some stage II patients are no longer receiving radiotherapy and lower total doses are being tried in both stage II and stage III cases. Shorter courses of chemotherapy are also being tried. The results of these new approaches have yet to be evaluated but so far the survival rates continue to improve.

The management of primarily inoperable tumours and of stage IV and stage V nephroblastoma continues to pose problems. General principles of good treatment must be applied but there is probably a necessity for some individualisation if the best results are to be achieved. These patients more than all others benefit from treatment in specialised centres. It is only in these centres, where the whole team has experience with large numbers of patients, that full evaluation of the patient can be carried out and the various permutations can be assessed.

In the case of tumours judged to be inoperable because of their size, treatment with cytotoxic drugs almost always reduces the bulk of the tumours and renders them resectable. There is no indication for heroic and life-threatening surgery in these patients. Ultrasonography or CT scanning may be of use in these children to follow the progress of the tumour during chemotherapy and to decide when operation is feasible. Most of these tumours will be resectable within 6 weeks of starting drugs. The small number who do not respond should receive 1,000−1,500 cGy of radiation but this should only be used when chemotherapy has failed because of the problems associated with large field radiation in such young patients.

In patients with stage IV disease, if the primary tumour is operable there is no known advantage in delaying nephrectomy unless the lung metastases are so large or have caused the development of pleural effusions so that anaesthesia may be hazardous and postoperative recovery complicated. Each patient should therefore be individually assessed and treatment given accordingly.

Before the regular use of chemotherapy about 15% of children with lung metastases were cured by pulmonary irradiation. There are several reports of children with lung metastases who have been cured with chemotherapy and it is debatable whether these patients should be given pulmonary irradiation and chemotherapy concurrently. The three drugs used, vincirstine, actinomycin D and adriamycin all enhance the effects of radiation. The cardiotoxicity of adriamycin is well documented so that the doses of radiation previously shown not to be associated with a risk of pneumonitis no longer apply and great care must be taken. Some authors have suggested chemotherapy followed by irradiation only if there is not complete regression of disease within a limited period of time. Others have advocated surgery for residual disease. It is again very much a decision to be based on the findings in the individual patient. Liver metastases are more difficult to treat and less responsive to available therapy. If they are detected before operation by ultrasound or scan it is worth trying preoperative chemotherapy to see whether regression can be obtained and in this case residual disease may become resectable. In patients with liver metastases, the liver must be subsequently included in the radiation field and care must be taken to monitor carefully for toxicity as the incidence of hepatopathy is increased by chemotherapy.

Bilateral nephroblastoma also requires individual assessment. Some patients will be amenable to primary surgery with bilateral partial nephrectomy or unilateral nephrectomy and contralateral partial nephrectomy. In other patients chemotherapy may be the best first treatment and may render inoperable tumours amenable to resection. Whether or not subsequent radiotherapy should be used will depend on the stage of the disease in each kidney. Some authorities have carried out bilateral nephrectomy and maintained the patient on chronic dialysis concurrent to chemotherapy, carrying out delayed renal transplantation when the risk of recurrence is past.

Follow-up

When the initial treatment has been completed regular careful follow-up of these patients is essential. All the multi-drug chemotherapy programmes described are associated with myelotoxicity and immune suppression. Regular chest x-rays should be done at 6-weekly intervals for the first 6 months and then at 3-monthly intervals to the end of the second year. They can then be done at lenghtening intervals. Renal function should also be checked, for although the remaining kidney is only occasionally in the radiation field the intensive drug treatment may well cause damage.

Long Term Effects

The long term effects of intensive treatment in young children must not be underestimated and all the patients treated in this way need prolonged observation.

Any area included in the radiation field is likely to suffer some interference with normal growth. This is why it essential that whole vertebrae are irradiated to prevent the development of scoliosis. Irradiation of one side of the pelvis will lead to differential growth. When it is necessary to irradiate the whole abdomen, even with careful shielding of the femoral heads there is some scatter of the radiation, and slipping of the femoral epiphyses is common.

Irradiation of the abdomen for Wilms' tumour usually includes the ovaries and a high proportion of female patients are sterile. They are probably best treated with hormone replacement to produce menstrual withdrawal bleeding. Boys may receive sufficient scattered radiation to the testes to cause oligozoospermia, but impotence has not been reported.

Table 2. Survival over successive 5-year intervals of 129 children with nephroblastoma treated in Manchester

Years	No. of patients	No. of survivors	% survivors
1954–1958	22	6	27
1959–1963	26	10	38
1964–1968	28	13	46
1969–1973	28	21	75
1974–1978	25	21	84

Osteomas are common in bones within the radiation field and a proportion of these may undergo malignant change. Other second primary neoplasms have also been reported. Late pneumonitis, hepatopathy and chronic nephritis have all been documented. Most of these patients were treated before the cumulative effects of combined treatment and the susceptibility of the growing child to them were so well recognised. As survival rates are now so good it is all the more important to be constantly vigilant for both short and long term problems associated with the management of these children.

Conclusions

The present treatment of nephroblastoma is one of the best examples of the effectiveness of a multidisciplinary approach. Such an approach has changed the outlook for more than 80% of children with this tumour. The increasing survival rates for all children treated in Manchester during successive five-year intervals from 1954 to 1978 are shown in Table 2. With careful assessment and the cooperation of surgeons, radiotherapists and chemo-therapists the future looks hopeful even for the remaining 20%.

References

1. Annotations (1877) Extirpation of the kidney. Lancet 1: 889
2. Barakat AY, Papadopoulou ZL, Chandra RS, Hollermann CE, Calcagro PL (1974) Pseudohermaphroditism, nephron disorder and Wilms tumour – a unifying concept. Paediatrics 54: 366–369
3. Beckwith JM (1970) Mesenchymal renal neoplasms of infancy (Editorial) J Paediatr Surg 5: 405–406
4. Beckwith JB (1974) Mesenchymal renal neoplasias of infancy revisited. J Paediatr Surg 9: 803–805
5. Beckwith JB, Palmer N (1978) Histopathology and prognosis of Wilms tumour. Cancer 41: 1937–1948
6. Bolande RP (1974a) Congenital mesoblastic nephroma. Arch Pathol 98: 357
7. Bolande RP (1974b) Congenital and infantile neoplasia of the kidney. Lancet 2: 1497–1499
8. Coley WB (1935) Wilms' tumour. Am J Surg 29: 463–464
9. D'Angio GJ, Evans AE, Breslow N (1976) The treatment of Wilms' tumour – results of the National Wilms' Tumour Study. Cancer 38: 633–646
10. D'Angio GJ, Beckwith JB, Breslow N, Sinks L, Sutow N, Wolff J (1979) Results of the Second National Wilms Tumour Study (NWTS-2). Proc Am Soc Clin Cancer (Abstr) 20: 309

11. Farber S, Toch R, Sears EM, Pinkel D (1956) Advances in chemotherapy of cancer in man. In: Greenstein JP, Haddew A (eds) Advances in cancer research, vol 4. Academic Press, New York, pp 1–71
12. Farewell VT, D'Angio GT, Breslow N, Norkool P (1981) Retrospective validation of a new staging system for Wilms' tumour. Cancer Clin Trials 4: 167–171
13. Friedlander A (1916) Sarcoma of the kidney treated by the roentgen ray. Am J Dis Child 12: 328–330
14. Ladda R, Atkins L, Littlefield J, Neurath P, Marimutha M (1974) Computer-assisted analysis of chromosomal abnormalities: detection of a deletion in aniridia-Wilms' tumour syndrome. Science 185: 784–788
15. Lemerle J, Voute PA, Tournade MP, Delemarre JFM, Jereb B, Ahstrom L, Flamant R, Gerard-Marchant R (1976) Preoperative versus postoperative radiotherapy, single versus multiple course of actinomycin D in the treatment of Wilms' tumour. Cancer 38: 647–659
16. Marsden HB, Lawler W (1978) Bone metastasising renal tumour of childhood. Br J Cancer 38: 437–441
17. Marsden HB, Lawler W (1980) Bone metastasising renal tumour of childhood. Virchows Archiv' [Pathol Anat] 387: 341–351
18. Morris Jones PH, Pearson D, Johnson AJ (1978) Management of nephroblastoma in childhood. Arch Dis Child 53: 112–119
19. Morse BS, Nussbaum M (1967) The detection of hyaluronic acid in the serum and urine of a patient. Am J Med 42: 996–1002
20. Wilms, M (1899) Die Mischgeschwülste der Nieren. Arthur Georgi, Leipsiz, pp 1–90
21. Wolff JA, Krivit W, Newton WA, D'Angio GJ (1968) Single versus multiple dose D-actinomycin therapy of Wilms' tumour. N Engl J Med 279: 290–294

Malignant Bone Tumors

J. A. Bullimore

Bristol Radiotherapy and Oncology Centre, Horfield Road, Bristol BS2 8ED, United Kingdom

Incidence

The annual incidence of cancer in children varies from country to country. The Manchester Tumour Register shows an incidence of 100 per million children under 15 years of age, whereas in the United States the Third National Cancer Survey conducted over the three year period 1969–1971 showed an annual incidence of 125 cases per million. Primary cancers of bone are uncommon and represent about 5%–6% of tumours occurring in children, the two most common forms being osteosarcoma and Ewing's sarcoma. Osteosarcoma is rare in children under the age of 5 years but its incidence rises rapidly during adolescence to reach a peak at about the age of 16 years. Ewing's tumour is seen more commonly than osteosarcoma in children under 10 years and it too increases in incidence with age to reach a peak in the late teens. In a review of bone tumours from the Mayo Clinic (Dahlin and Coventry 1967) it was reported that of 530 malignant primary bone tumours, there were 294 osteosarcomas in patients aged between 10 and 20 years and only 25 in patients aged under 10 years, whereas there were 103 Ewing's tumours in patients aged between 10 and 20 years and 45 in patients aged under 10 years.
Other bone tumours are rare in childhood and include fibrosarcoma, reticulum cell sarcoma (lymphoma of bone), chondrosarcoma, parosteal osteosarcoma, giant cell tumour, haemangioendothelioma and haemangiopericytoma.

Presenting Features

The commonest presenting features are pain and swelling. Occasionally pathological fracture may occur or attention may be drawn to the tumour by a relatively minor injury. Rarely the presentation is accompanied by a fever.

Osteosarcoma

Osteosarcoma in most series is slightly more common in males than in females and tends to occur in the metaphyses of long bones. The majority of tumours occur in the distal femur, 90% of all osteosarcomas being in the region of the knee. Diagnosis is made by means of a biopsy. X-ray examination usually shows destruction of the bone with loss of the normal trabecular pattern and new bone formation. There is considerable variation in the x-ray appearances but characteristically sun-ray spicules of new bone formation and a Codman's triangle are present and frequently there is massive extension into the soft tissues. The

Recent Results in Cancer Research. Vol. 88
© Springer-Verlag Berlin · Heidelberg 1983

alkaline phosphatase level is usually raised. Following diagnosis, the extent of the disease within the bone is ascertained with conventional tomograms and, when possible, computerised tomography (CT) scans. X-ray and CT scan of the chest and an isotope skeletal survey are performed to detect lung and bone metastases.

Clinical Course

Osteosarcoma disseminates via the blood stream and most commonly gives rise to pulmonary metastases. Infrequently, lymphatic spread to regional nodes occurs. Spread to other bones is usually not manifest until metastases in the lungs have been established for some time and perhaps represents tertiary spread from the lung secondaries. Before the use of modern methods of treatment 80% of patients had developed lung metastases within 2 years of presentation and the survival at 5 years in most series was less than 20%.

Management of Osteosarcoma with No Metastases

Until recently the modern treatment of choice for primary tumours of long bones was amputation or disarticulation of the limb followed by adjuvant chemotherapy. First reports of favourable responses to high dose methotrexate and adriamycin used as an adjuvant in the treatment of osteosarcoma first appeared in 1974 when Jaffe et al. reported increases in survival rates using high dose methotrexate in the order of $1-2\,g/m^2$ together with vincristine. In 1977 Cortes et al. published the results of using adriamycin as adjuvant chemotherapy. Since that time numerous schedules of chemotherapy have been used in various studies mainly in the United States but also in Europe and Britain. Most of the studies have included adriamycin and high dose methotrexate, the dose of methotrexate sometimes reaching 10 or more g/m^2. Combinations of bleomycin, cyclophosphamide, dimethyl triazeno imidazole carboxamide (DTIC) and more recently *cis*-platinum have been employed. Most of the studies undertaken have included relatively small numbers of patients due to the rarity of the disease. What is important is that when the literature is reviewed there is a remarkable uniformity in the results (Tables 1 and 2).
A large trial of adjuvant therapy in osteosarcoma in long bones has recently been completed in Britain by the Medical Research Council (MRC). Low dose methotrexate ($200\,mg/m^2$) as a bolus injection plus vincristine was given every 3 weeks, and compared with similar chemotherapy alternating 3-weekly with adriamycin. The study has now been closed with an entry of 200 patients but the results have not yet been published. It is expected that the results will not differ greatly from other published results.
The European Organisation for Research and Treatment of Cancer (EORTC) is currently running a study in which it is aimed to enter 400 patients. The adjuvant therapy is randomised between three arms. The first arm comprises chemotherapy alone using high dose methotrexate ($6\,g/m^2$) as an infusion over 6 hours with folinic acid rescue, alternating every 2 weeks with adriamycin for 9 weeks; then cyclophosphamide is added 2 weeks after the adriamycin to complete a 6-week cycle which is repeated six times. The second arm of the trial consists of whole lung irradiation, 2,000 cGy in 10 fractions over 2 weeks to the whole of both lungs using cobalt-60 radiation. The third arm consists of chemotherapy for 9 weeks as in the first arm, followed by radiotherapy to the whole of both lungs given as in the second arm. No further chemotherapy is given. The results of this study are not yet

Table 1. Comparison of the resuls of different regimes of adjuvant chemotherapy in the treatment of patients with osteosarcoma

Investigators	Adjuvant treatment	% disease-free survival		
		2 years	3 years	5 years
Jaffe et al. (1978)	HDMTX	42	–	–
Sutow et al. (1978)	CONPADRI I[b]			
	COMPARDI II	50	–	–
	COMPADRI III			
Cortes et al. (1978)	Adriamycin	–	–	40[a]
Cortes et al. (1979)	Adriamycin	–	48[a]	–
Cortes et al. (1981)	Adriamycin + HDMTX	–	34[a]	–
Rosenberg et al. (1979)	HDMTX	38[a]	–	–
Ettinger et al. (1980)	Adriamycin + cis-platinum	58[a]	–	–

[a] Life table estimates
[b] See Table 2

Table 2. Comparison of the combination chemotherapy regimes

Drug	Conpadri I	Compadri II	Compadri III
Vincristine (No. of doses)	12	15	14
Cyclophosphamide	10 mg/kg/day × 7 for 3 courses	Same	Same
Adriamycin (cumulative dose)	390 mg/m^2	120 mg/m^2	360 mg/m^2
Melphalan	0.3 mg/kg for 4 pulses	0.3 mg/kg for 4 pulses	0.3 mg/kg for 3 pulses
Methotrexate	None	3 pulses (75 mg, 100 mg, 150 mg/kg)	3 pulses (75 mg, 150 mg, 200 mg/kg)

The periodicity of giving the cytotoxic agents is very different in the three regimes

published, but are not expected to show major differences from other reported studies.

The present position of adjuvant chemotherapy in the management of osteosarcoma is that various regimes using widely differing doses of drugs, in particular a wide range of methotrexate dosage, appear to give very similar results at 2-year true follow-up (rather than by projected results based on life-tables). It has not yet been proved that adjuvant chemotherapy increases the cure rate but the fact that it increases the survival rate of those patients studied probably means a true increase in cure rate is also achieved. Recurrences as late as 5 years from treatment make assessment of cure difficult.

Attempts to relate treatment to tumour response are now being made. Preoperative chemotherapy enables assessment to be made of the degree of necrosis achieved in the resected tumour. In 1981, Rosen et al. reported the results of "T-7" and "T-10" protocols, and these have attracted a good deal of attention. A total of 93 patients were treated with preoperative chemotherapy (T-7) consisting of high dose methotrexate, adriamyin and bleomycin, cyclophosphamide and DTIC (BCD). Forty-nine patients showed a histologically favourable response; T-7 chemotherapy was continued postoperatively, and 48 of these patients remained disease-free with a median follow-up of 31 months. Of the remaining 44 patients, 15 continued on the same chemotherapeutic regime as had been given preoperatively and ten had developed metastases by a median time of 13 months. Twenty-nine patients whose tumours did not show a good histological response received a regime of *cis*-platinum, adriamycin and BCD (T-10) postoperatively. Twenty-seven patients (93%) were disease-free with a median follow-up of 18 months. These figures must be viewed with caution as very short term results are likely to be misleading as has proved to be the case in other premature publications.

Limb Preservation

In the past few years there have been increasing attempts to save the affected limb by means of prosthetic replacement of the involved bone. Encouraging results obtained with the use of adjuvant chemotherapy and the management of metastatic disease of the lungs using chemotherapy and surgery have led to a policy of resecting the tumour and reconstructing the limb using a prosthetic replacement for the bone. Intensive preoperative chemotherapy is used and in some cases may continue for as long as 12 or more weeks before surgery. Assessment of the response of the primary tumour to chemotherapy is made before surgery by means of repeated isotope bone scans and measurements of serum alkaline phosphatase. In a favourable response, the uptake of isotope at the site of the tumour may be shown to be reduced and alkaline phosphatase levels falls. Clinicians at the Memorial Hospital in New York have been pioneers in this method of treatment and similar studies are now being undertaken in Great Britain. Previously, lesions of the humerus were thought to be most suitable for prosthetic replacement but now suitable prostheses are being used for lower limbs. Remarkably good functional results can be obtained. In selected patients given intensive chemotherapy before resection successful control of local tumours is achieved in the majority of cases. Regimes used in the Bristol Royal Infirmary, working in conjunction with Mr. Rodney Sneath of the Royal Orthopaedic Hospital, Birmingham, consist of high dose methotrexate given as an infusion over 8 hours with folinic acid rescue and preceded by vincristine. Methotrexate is given weekly, escalating the dose to a maximum of 6 g/m^2 and surgery undertaken between 3 and 6 weeks from the start of the chemotherapy. Two weeks after surgery, chemotherapy is restarted using a 4-week cycle with vincristine and high ose methotrexate (in the highest dose which had been tolerated by the patient before surgery) on day 1 and adriamycin on day 7. Treatment is continued for 1 year after the operation.

Management of Patients with Lung Metastases

Nowadays, lung metastases from an osteosarcoma are most common in patients who have previously received radical treatment including adjuvant chemotherapy for the primary lesions. This may necessitate modification of subsequent chemotherapy. When a patient is found to have lung metastases careful assessment is carried out to ascertain whether there are metastases elsewhere and whether the primary tumour is under control, in which case plans are made to remove the lung metastases. Careful assessment of the size and distribution of the lesions are made with CT scans of the whole lungs. If bilateral metastases are present two thoracotomies are planned with a gap of approximately six weeks. Multiple lung metastases are removed by multiple wedge resections. Occasionally, if larger metastases are present, partial or total lobectomy may be employed. Lung function studies are undertaken and the surgeon must be convinced that, following removal of the necessary amount of lung together with the tumour, the patient will still have adequate respiratory function. Before surgery, chemotherapy as described for prosthetic replacement of the primary tumour is undertaken. Methotrexate is given weekly for 3–4 weeks before thoracotomy with the dose escalating from $1 \, g/m^2$ to $4 \, g/m^2$. Surgery is undertaken approximately 7–10 days after the last preoperative methotrexate infusion and chemotherapy is restarted approximately 10 days after surgery. Particular caution must be used however, in restarting high dose methotrexate as it must be ensured that there is no residual pleural effusion postoperatively. Such an effusion could act as a reservoir for the methotrexate and lead to severe toxicity. Therefore whenever possible adriamycin is used as the first agent postoperatively and 2–3 weeks later the cycle of high dose methotrexate (in the maximum dose tolerated by the patient preoperatively) on day 1 and adriamycin on day 7 is started in a 4-week cycle for 12 months. However, if the patient has previously received the maximum tolerable dose of adriamycin in a previous course of adjuvant therapy or when the maximum cumulative dose of adriamycin has been given, it is discontinued and high dose methotrexate is given 3-weekly.

Between 1976 and 1981 fourteen patients with lung metastases arising from osteosarcoma were treated using the Bristol protocol of vincristine and high dose methotrexate, with or without adriamycin followed by removal of lung metastases. One of these patients had pulmonary metastases present at the time of first presentation. The rest developed metastases following successful treatment of the primary tumour. Ten patients had unilateral disease and four patients had bilateral metastases. In seven patients pulmonary metastases recurred and repeat thoracotomy was done for these. Life table analysis of the results show a 3-year survival rate of 48%. However, this level is probably falsely high due to the short length of follow-up on some of the patients and the small number of patients included in the study. However, two patients in the series have survived without disease for more than 5 years after the last of their thoracotomies.

Management of Patients with Other Than Bony Metastases

Patients who have multiple bony metastases have not been successfully treated by chemotherapy. It is very doubtful whether aggressive chemotherapy should be undertaken in such patients, who have, by the nature of their disease, a very short time to live. Their management is probably best restricted to radiotherapy for pain relief and other symptomatic treatment. Similarly, if there are lung metastases of such a number and in a site not amenable to resection it is again doubtful if aggressive treatment with chemotherapy should be undertaken.

Developments in the Management of Osteosarcoma

The problem that has beset studies of patients with osteosarcoma has been that most of the reported results are of groups of patients which are too small to give statistically significant results. However, an overall trend towards increased survival of patients with osteosarcoma has been observed since the introduction of adjuvant chemotherapy in the early 1970s and the development of more aggressive management of pulmonary metastatic disease. In studies of patients treated before 1970 the 5-year survival rate was around 20%, but rates for centres employing more aggressive methods of treatment have improved markedly. In Bristol the rate has reached 46% and similar results have been achieved in a number of American and European centres.

A controversy has arisen because of the uniformity of results reported in studies of adjuvant therapy. It has been suggested that the natural history of the disease may have altered and that the results of treating the primary tumour by ablation alone might compare favourably with those reported following the addition of adjuvant chemotherapy. The Mayo Clinic in America is currently running a randomised study in which cytotoxic chemotherapy is either given soon after treatment of the primary tumour or delayed until metastases occur. A recent interim analysis indicates that the 2-year survival curves of the two treatment groups in the study are similar.

The only way to ascertain the competence and usefulness of chemotherapy and other methods of treatment of patients with osteosarcoma is by undertaking large studies. This can only be achieved by cooperation between centres. It would appear that increasing the aggressiveness of postoperative chemotherapy is unlikely to significantly affect survival rates. It is therefore being suggested that preoperative chemotherapy, possibly for 2–3 months, should be given to all patients, not only those who are suitable for limb preservation techniques. It is hoped that such a study will be undertaken jointly by the EORTC and the MRC in the near future.

The outlook for patients with osteosarcoma has improved markedly with regard to prolonged survival since the early 1970s, but the improvement in long term cure is not so great. The quality of life for an increasing proportion of patients is being greatly improved by the development of successful surgical techniques for internal prostheses and limb preservation.

Ewing's Sarcoma

Ewing's sarcoma is a highly malignant tumour which had a cure rate of only about 10% before the use of chemotherapy was introduced (Nesbit 1976). Following presentation of the patient the extent of the local and metastatic disease must first be established, exactly as described for patients with osteosarcoma. Ewing's sarcoma does not have such an overwhelming tendency to occur in the long bones as osteosarcoma does; it often arises in the spine, pelvis and shoulder girdles and on rare occasions in the skull. In many sites ablative surgery is not possible. The use of radiotherapy may achieve local tumour control, the probability of control being related to the dose given. A dose of 6,000 cGy given in daily fractions over 6 weeks, or the radiobiological equivalent in different treatment schedules, is required (Rosen et al. 1976). Treatment of the whole of the tumour-bearing bone is desirable but not always possible. In children, if a long bone is being treated the epiphysis furthest from the lesion can often be spared provided that a large margin of apparently normal bone separates it from the tumour. In this way stunting of bone growth may be lessened. When using a dose of 6,000 cGy, 4,000 cGy in 4 weeks are given to the "whole" bone and a further 2,000 cGy in 2 weeks to a smaller volume which includes the tumour and a 2 cm margin surrounding it.

In treating limbs where a good functional result is the aim, care must be taken not to treat the limbs circumferentially and to leave a strip of untreated soft tissue at least 3 cm wide over the whole length of the irradiated volume. This procedure prevents the occurrence of a tight band of fibrosis in the treated area encircling the limb, and distal oedema is thus avoided. Megavoltage apparatus must always be employed. There must be good immobilisation of the part to be treated and tissue compensators where necessary should be used. Each field should be treated daily and treatment should not be started until the biopsy wound is healed. When tumours occur in bones where removal would not result in severe functional loss or deformity, radical excision may sometimes be successful, for example in the head of the fibula. However, as there is frequently a large soft tissue component, such excisions are rarely feasible.

The development of successful internal prostheses may make surgery a more acceptable method of primary treatment in some patients. Young children with Ewing's sarcoma present a particular problem of local control, as limb irradiation will result in loss of limb growth. If the lesion is in the lower limb amputation may be the best local treatment. The use of internal prostheses in very young children cannot yet overcome the problem of unacceptable limb shortening as the child gets older. An important role for surgery lies in removal of residual bulk tumour following radiotherapy and chemotherapy. This can be illustrated by the case of a 14-year-old boy with a massive tumour arising in the right pubic bone with gross soft tissue involvement. Following chemotherapy and radical radiotherapy to the hemipelvis there was marked shrinkage of the tumour but on CT scan a mass was still visible, impinging on the bladder. Surgery was undertaken and the pubic bone and attached mass were removed. A good gait has been preserved with minimal deformity. It will be necessary to continue chemotherapy postoperatively for approximately 18 months.

As in osteosarcoma the main problem to overcome is the development of metastases. Local control of the tumour can usually be achieved by radiotherapy with or without surgery, except where the lesions are in a site where radical excision or radical doses of radiotherapy are not possible.

Chemotherapy has a vital role to play in the cure of Ewing's tumour and it must be used whether or not the local treatment consists of radiation or of surgery. Metastases occur early in the natural history of the tumour and for this reason chemotherapy must be started as soon as diagnosis is established and staging has been completed. Vincristine, actinomycin D, cyclophosphamide and adriamycin used in combination have been shown to be effective in Ewing's tumour (Rosen 1976). The United Kingdom Children's Cancer Study Group (UKCCSG) has been carrying out such a study since 1978 in which one cycle of vincristine, cyclophosphamide and adriamycin (VCAd) is given before the start of radiation therapy. Reduced doses of vincristine and cyclophosphamide are given weekly throughout radiotherapy, and on its completion vincristine, actinomycin D and cyclophosphamide (VAC) alternate with VCAd every 3 weeks to complete 2 years. Early results of this study are encouraging, with prolonged survival already demonstrable.

Treatment of Patients with Lung Metastases

Lung metastases from Ewing's tumour are most likely to be multiple and are usually not suitable for surgical resecting. By combining lung irradiation and chemotherapy, cure may still be achieved. Repeated courses of VAC/VCAd are given to produce some shrinkage of the lesion (usually three or four courses). Whole lung irradiation to a dose of 1,500 cGy in 2 weeks using megavoltage is given and an additional 1,000 cGy using narrow "pencil beam" radiation fields is added locally to any residual lesions still demonstrable by CT scan. Chemotherapy is recommenced 10–14 days after irradiation; the dose during the first course is half that given in the initial period of treatment and prednisolone is added to reduce the incidence of "radiation-recall" pneumonitis. In subsequent courses full doses can usually be given and prednisolone may no longer to be needed. The adriamycin is omitted after radiotherapy to the thorax, due to increased risk of adriamycin cardiomyopathy.

Treatment of Patients with Bone Metastases

In Ewing's sarcoma, spread to other bones occurs more frequently than in osteosarcoma. At present, cure of Ewing's sarcoma with bony metastases is not possible but pain relief can often be achieved using local radiotherapy. Chemotherapy in these circumstances is not always appropriate, but systemic treatment with whole body irradiation, with an initial dose of 600 cGy in a single exposure to the upper or lower half of the body, followed 6 weeks later by a similar dose to the other half of the body, can produce good and sometimes prolonged palliation with minimal morbidity.

Conclusions

Although the progress towards cure of the majority of children with bone sarcoma is slow, in the last decade improvements in both survival rates and quality of life have been achieved.

References

1. Cortes EP, Holland JF, Wang JJ, Glidewell O (1977) Amputation and adriamycin (ADM) in primary osteosarcoma (OS). A preliminary report. Proc Am Assoc Cancer Res/Proc Am Soc Clin Oncol 18: 297–298
2. Cortes EP, Holland JF, Glidewell O (1978) Amputation and adriamycin in primary osteosarcoma. A 5-year report. Cancer Treat Rep 62: 271–277
3. Cortes EP, Necheles TF, Holland JF, Glidewell O (1979) Adriamycin (ADM) alone versus ADM and high dose methotrexate citrovorum factor rescue (HDMTX-CF) as adjuvant to operable primary osteosarcoma (OS): a randomized study by Cancer and Leukaemia Group B (CALGB). Proc Am Assoc Cancer Res/Proc Am Soc Clin Oncol (Abstr C-498) 20: 412
4. Cortes EP, Wenberg V, Holland JF, Carey RW for the CALGB (1981) Adjuvant chemotherapy with adriamycin for primary osteosarcoma. Proc Am Assoc Cancer Res/Proc Am Soc Clin Oncol (Abstr C-280) 22: 404
5. Dahlin DC, Coventry MB (1967) Osteogenic sarcoma: a study of six hundred cases. J Bone Joint Surg 49: 101–110
6. Ettinger LJ, Douglass HO Jr, Higby DJ, Nime F, Mindell ER, Ghoorah J, Sinks LF, Freeman AI (1980) Adriamycin (ADR) and *cis*-diamminedichloroplatinum (DDP) as adjuvant therapy in osteosarcoma of the extremities. Proc Am Assoc Cancer Res/Proc Am Soc Clin Oncol (Abstr C-292) 21: 392
7. Jaffe N, Frei E III, Traggis D, Bishop Y (1974) Adjuvant methotrexate and citrovorum factor treatment of osteogenic sarcoma. N Engl J Med 291: 994–997
8. Jaffe N, Frei E III, Watts H, Traggis D (1978) High-dose methotrexate in osteogenic sarcoma: a 5-year experience. Cancer Treat Rep 62: 259–264

9. Nesbit ME (1976) Ewing's sarcoma. CA 26: 176–181
10. Rosen G (1976) Management of malignant bone tumours in children and adolescents. Pediatr Clin North Am 23: 183–213
11. Rosen G, Huvos M, Nirenberg A, Caparros B (1981) Osteogenic sarcoma (OS): selection of adjuvant chemotherapy (CT) based upon the response of the primary tumour to preoperative (PreO) CT. Proc Am Assoc Cancer Res/Proc Am Soc Clin Oncol (Abstr C-378) 22: 429
12. Rosenberg SA, Chabner BA, Young RC, Clippca (1979) Treatment of osteogenic sarcoma. 1. Effect of adjuvant high dose methotrexate after amputation. Cancer Treat Rep 63: 739–751
13. Sutow WW, Gehan EA, Dyment PC, Vietti T, Miale T (1978) Multidrug adjuvant chemotherapy for osteosarcoma. Interim report of the Southwest Oncology Group Studies. Cancer Treat Rep 62: 265–269

Soft Tissue Sarcomas in Children

J. S. Malpas*

Imperial Cancer Research Fund Department of Medical Oncology, St. Bartholomew's Hospital, London EC1A 7BE, United Kingdom

Introduction

Soft tissue sarcomas occur throughout childhood. By far the commonest is rhabdomyosarcoma, but undifferentiated embryonal sarcomas, fibrosarcomas, liposarcomas and synovial sarcomas may occur. Rhabdomyosarcoma accounts for more than 10% of childhood malignant solid tumours, and was seen in 11.3% of 612 successive children treated by the Royal Marsden Hospital and St Bartholomew's Hospital Children's Solid Tumour Group. It is being used as a model for development of treatment of other soft tissue sarcomas, and it will form the main subject of this chapter.

Rhabdomyosarcoma

This highly malignant tumour occurs with approximately equal frequency in both sexes throughout childhood. The embryonal form of the disease occurs more often in younger children, and the alveolar histological appearance is seen most commonly in the young adolescent. The distribution of the disease is worldwide, but it affects black children three times less frequently than white. No familial associations are apparent, but a definite link has been found between carcinoma of the breast on the maternal side of the family and incidence of rhabdomyosarcoma in the children (Li and Fraumeni 1979).

Pathology

The tumours are soft fleshy pink or grey-pink masses which readily infiltrate along tissue planes. Histological appearance is described as embryonal, alveolar, botryoid or pleomorphic. The rhabdomyoblast contains glycogen and sometimes muscle striations, which can be stained using the phosphotungstic acid method. Electron microscopy may aid diagnosis by showing the characteristic cytoplasmic fibrils. Pleomorphic rhabdomyosarcoma is very rarely seen in childhood.

---

* The patients presented in this report have been under the care of Dr. J. E. Freeman, Dr. J. Graham-Pole and Dr. E. R. Sandland. Dr. A. G. Stansfeld has been responsible for the histological diagnosis, and I have been much helped by Dr. J. Kingston in reviewing the data. Mr D. Hughes of the Research Centre for Mathematical Modelling of Clinical Trials at Warwick University has provided the actuarial curves. I am grateful to Jo Barton for typing the manuscript

Recent Results in Cancer Research. Vol. 88
© Springer-Verlag Berlin · Heidelberg 1983

Staging

A number of staging classifications have been used for rhabdomyosarcoma. In discussion of the results of the author's studies, the St Jude classification (Pratt et al. 1972) has been used (Table 1).

Clinical Features

Rhabdomyosarcoma presents with a slightly increased ratio of male to female patients. In 62 children with this condition seen at St Bartholomew's Hospital between 1956 and 1981, 34 were boys and 28 were girls, giving a male to female ratio of 1.2 : 1. The mean age of presentation was the same in both sexes — 5 years and 8 months.

The tumour may present in the orbit, extra-orbital sites in the head and neck, the thorax, intra-abdominal sites, the genitourinary tract or the extremities.

There is therefore a wide variety of clinical presentations. An example of this is seen in a current study of 62 children (Table 2). Of these, 47 had tumours presenting as soft tissue swellings. Pain was a major presenting feature in 22 children, and general symptoms such as malaise, fever and weight loss occurred in 17. A variety of other symptoms and signs included proptosis, double vision, dysuria, haematuria, vaginal bleeding and nasal discharge, depending on the site of presentation.

Staging based on the St Jude's criteria gave the distribution of presentation shown in Table 3. The majority of children at presentation have disease which is quite advanced. In

Table 1. St Jude Children's Research Hospital staging scheme

Stage I	Localised. Recognised tumour completely resected	
Stage II	Regional. Adjacent infiltration, local or regional lymph nodes involved	
	A.	Tumour completely resectable
	B.	Tumour non-resectable, or only partially
Stage III	Generalised	
	A.	Distant metastases with normal bone marrow
	B.	Distant metastases with bone marrow infiltration

Table 2. Sites of presentation of rhabdomyosarcoma in children in the St Bartholomew's study, 1956–1981

Site	No. of patients
Orbit	11
Head and neck	12
Thorax	6
Abdomen	2
Genitourinary tract	20
Limbs	7
Unknown primary site	4
Total	62

Table 3. Stage at presentation of rhabdomyosarcoma in the St Bartholomew's study

	No. of patients
Stage I	10
Stage IIA	10
IIB	30
Stage IIIA	5
IIIB	7
Total	62

Table 4. Site of presentation of rhabdomyosarcoma related to stage (St Bartholomews' study)

Site	Stage					
	I	IIA	IIB	IIIA	IIIB	Total
Orbit	2	2	7	0	0	11
Head and neck	0	2	10	0	0	12
Thorax	0	2	3	1	0	6
Abdomen	0	0	1	1	0	2
Genitourinary tract	4	3	8	3	2	20
Limbs	4	1	1	0	1	7
Disseminated	0	0	0	0	4	4
Total	10	10	30	5	7	62

reviewing the stage of children presenting in a large number of series, Green and Jaffe (1978) noted the frequency with which children with tumour of the head and neck had regional and unresectable disease. They also noted the frequency with which tumours of the trunk and extremities showed metastases at presentation.

In the present study the majority of children with head and neck tumours are clearly shown to be in the more advanced stage of the disease (Table 4). However, this study shows that tumours arising in the limbs have been detected at a relatively early stage.

Investigation

It is obviously not possible to define specific programmes of investigation for rhabdomyosarcoma, as its manifestations are so varied that the extent of investigation will depend on the site of occurrence and the apparent extent of disease. It will also depend to some extent on the treatment programme adopted. In the series reported, most children presenting from 1971 onwards had, in addition to routine investigation, a bone marrow examination and lymphography where appropriate. More recently, isotope scanning to detect bony metastases, and computerised axial tomography (CT) scanning to define the extent of disease have been used. All children in our series, on completion of therapy, have had the appropriate investigations repeated to define response.

Occult metastases in bone have been seen frequently in series of children who clinically appeared to have localised disease. Only in neuroblastoma is there greater frequency of bone marrow infiltration. Of 40 children in the current study who ostensibly had local disease only, bone marrow infiltration occurred in seven (17%). Isotope bone scanning proved to be useful, in that 13 (33%) of the 40 children had bone scans which demonstrated abnormal uptake of isotope. A positive bone scan was of considerable prognostic significance; of the 13 patients whose scans were positive only two survive.

CT scanning was chiefly used to define the extent of disease already suspected clinically, and confirmed a tumour in 75% of the patients investigated. An important finding was that, almost invariably, the scan revealed much more extensive disease than had been suspected by the clinical assessment.

Management

The results of treatment of rhabdomyosarcoma by radiotherapy or surgery alone have been disappointing, with an overall survival rate (i.e. for all treatments) of just over 10% (Pratt et al. 1972; Green and Jaffe 1978). Successful surgical excision or local irradiation of small primary tumours, though successful, was complicated in many cases by the occurrence of metastases in the lungs, bones and liver. With the introduction of actinomycin D, vincristine and cyclophosphamide, used either individually or in combination, temporary regression of these metastases was seen, but they soon recurred. Pinkel and Pickren (1961) first suggested that chemotherapy should be used at presentation in combination with radiotherapy or surgery for effective control of the primary tumour. They reported long term survival in a child with a rhabdomyosarcoma of the face. Pratt et al. (1972) reported the results treating 20 children with rhabdomyosarcoma with surgery, radiotherapy and adjuvant chemotherapy using vincristine, actinomycin D and cyclophosphamide. Fifteen children responded completely and of these, seven were tumour-free for up to 3 years. Successful therapy using these procedures has now been reported by many groups (Malpas et al. 1976; Maurer et al. 1977; Ransom and Pratt 1977; Malek and Kelalis 1977).

Many questions have been raised following these successful studies. In a preliminary report, Maurer et al. (1977), for the Intergroup Rhabdomyosarcoma Study, in which 433 children with previously untreated rhabdomyosarcoma were entered, showed that when local disease only was present, the addition of radiotherapy to the primary site of tumour after complete excision did not increase survival rate. When residual disease had been present, the use of three-drug rather than two-drug combination as adjuvant therapy was of no benefit. When metastatic disease had been present, the addition of adriamycin to the three-drug combination did not increase its effectiveness.

Where children have been available for assessment after chemotherapy without radiotherapy, Pratt and George (1980), using various combinations of vincristine, cyclophosphamide, actinomycin D and adriamycin, found that where the disease had not been eradicated by the initial surgery and was evaluable, chemotherapy did not always completely eliminate the tumour. Five out of 39 patients with stage IIB disease, and ten out of 17 with stage IIIB disease showed a complete response. Neither the age of the patient, the histological appearance of the tumour, its site, nor the chemotherapy programme used influenced the outcome.

The site of the primary disease has been shown to be of considerable importance in determining the outcome of treatment. In our review of 62 children very different survival rates were seen for patients with tumours arising in various sites (Fig. 1).

In 141 children with head and neck involvement, Tefft et al. (1978), reporting for the Intergroup Rhabdomyosarcoma Study, showed that of 54 patients with tumours in

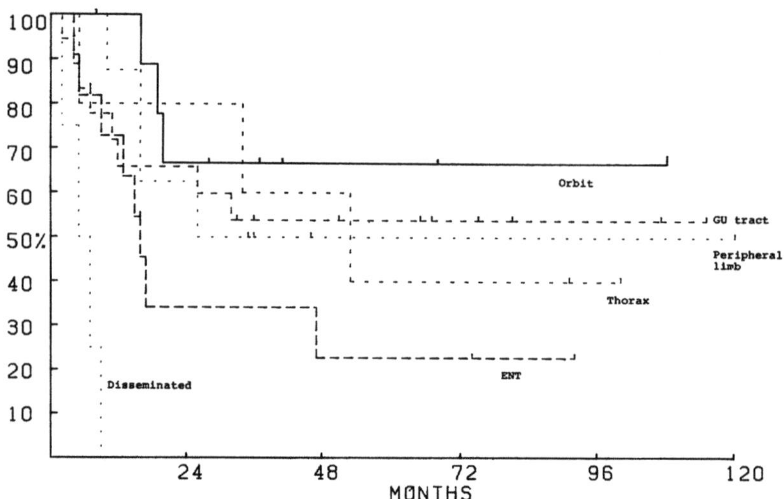

Fig. 1. Actuarial survival of children with rhabdomyosarcoma related to primary site of presentation

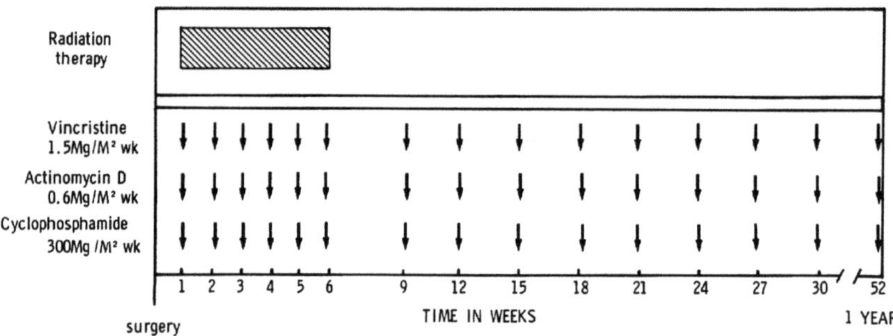

Fig. 2. Protocol I schedule for combination chemotherapy of childhood rhabdomyosarcoma which was used from 1973–1977, but no longer advised

parameningeal sites, 20 (35%) developed direct meningeal extensions, and 18 (90%) of these children died from this complication. Meningeal extension must be anticipated in children with tumours in parameningeal sites, and their radiotherapy planned to cover adjacent meninges. In view of this, neuraxis irradiation has been suggested, as chemotherapy does not seem to be effective in providing prophylaxis.

In 43 children treated with surgery, radiotherapy and chemotherapy on protocols I and II at St Bartholomew's Hospital (Figs. 2, 3, 4), the stage of the tumour was an important determinant of prognosis (Fig. 5). In studying the effect of stage on survival, it is notable that the effectiveness of the combination of radiotherapy and chemotherapy appears to reduce the prognostic significance of whether or not the local tumour was resectable. It has been suggested that, in a variety of solid tumours, the size of the initial tumour may influence outcome and be an important determinant for prognosis; this applies particularly to neuroblastoma and Ewing's tumour. With this in mind, the size of primary tumours in these 43 children was reviewed, and the children divided into three groups: those that presented with tumours of diameter less than 5 cm ("small" tumours), 5–15 cm ("large")

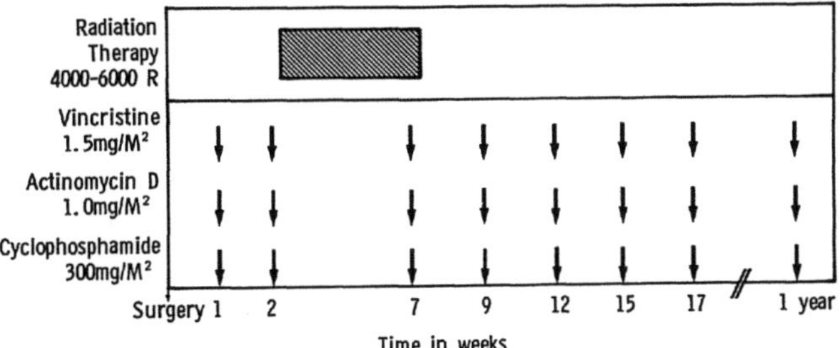

Fig. 3. Protocol II schedule for combination chemotherapy for "good prognosis" rhabdomyosarcoma, used from 1977

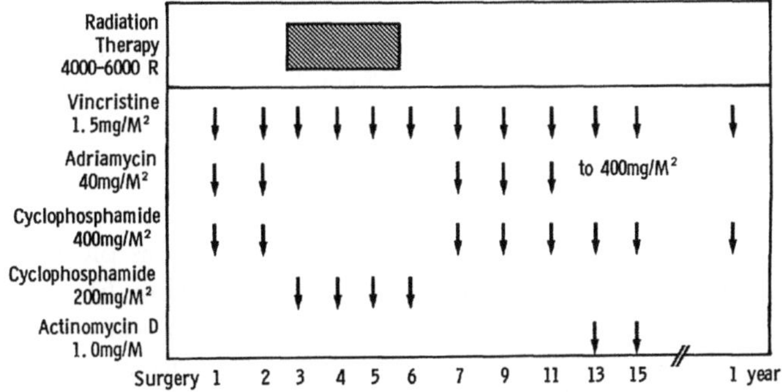

Fig. 4. Protocol II schedule for combination chemotherapy for "bad prognosis" rhabdomyosarcoma, used from 1977

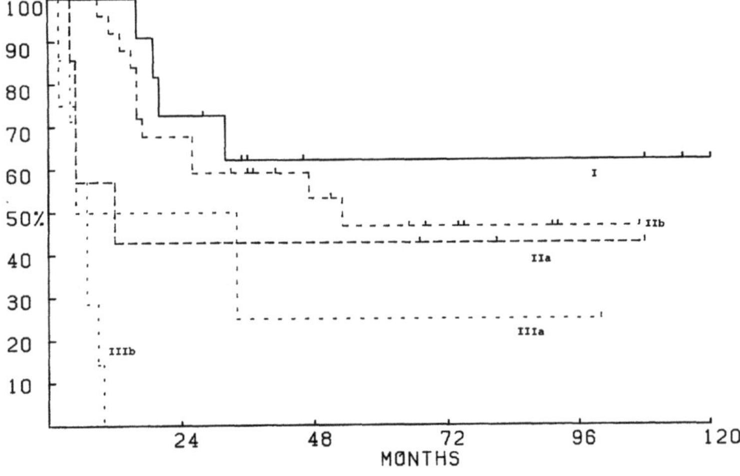

Fig. 5. Actuarial survival of children with rhabdomyosarcoma related to the stage, as assessed using the St. Jude criteria

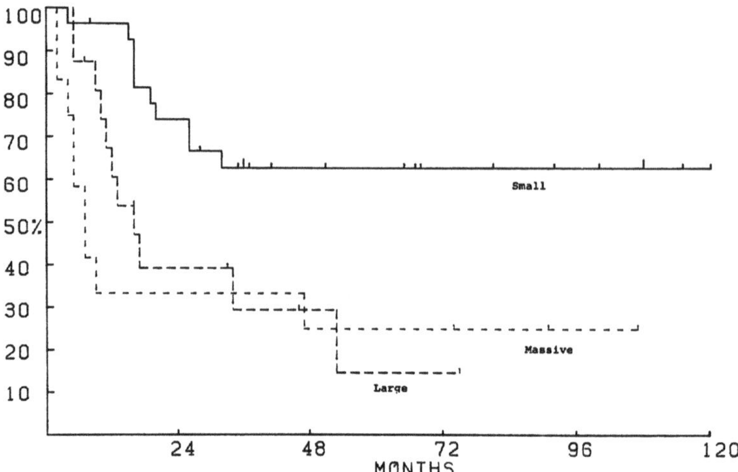

Fig. 6. Actuarial survival of children with rhabdomyosarcoma related to the size of the primary tumour at presentation (small, < 5 cm diameter; large, 5–15 cm diameter; and massive, > 15 cm diameter)

and over 16 cm ("massive"). When survival was plotted, it was seen to be significantly greater in the group with "small" tumours (Fig. 6).

Although there has been a considerable improvement in the outlook for children with rhabdomyosarcoma, the current therapy for disseminated tumour and tumour in specific sites such as head and neck is still unsatisfactory. Studies are now in progress to see whether further improvement in results can be achieved by the use of high dose combination chemotherapy followed by radiotherapy or surgery depending on the site and extent of residual tumour. An alternative possibility, involving treatment with very high dose chemotherapy and autologous bone marrow transplantation is also being investigated.

Conclusions

The presenting features, clinical findings, and results of investigation and treatment of 62 children with rhabdomyosarcoma, presenting consecutively at St Bartholomew's Hospital, have been described. The site of presentation of disease, the stage of the disease and the size of the primary tumour appear to be major determinants of prognosis. A combined approach to therapy, utilising surgery, radiotherapy and chemotherapy, has resulted in a significant improvement in survival and cure rates. However, for some children, with disseminated disease, or with disease in primary sites such as the head and neck, the prognosis is still poor, new treatment programmes designed to deal with these problems are being investigated.

References

1. Green DM, Jaffe N (1978) Progress and controversy in the treatment of childhood rhabdomyosarcoma. Cancer Treat Rev 5: 7–23
2. Li FP, Fraumeni JF (1979) Soft tissue sarcomas, breast cancer and other neoplasms. A familial syndrome? Ann Intern Med 71: 747–752
3. Malek RS, Kelalis PP (1977) Paratesticular rhabdomyosarcoma in childhood. J Urol 118: 450–453
4. Malpas JS, Freeman JE, Paxton AM, Walker-Smith J, Stansfeld AG, Wood CBS (1976) Radiotherapy and adjuvant combination chemotherapy for childhood rhabdomyosarcoma. Br Med J 1: 247–249
5. Maurer HM, Moon I, Donaldson M, Fernandez C, Gehan EA, Hammond D, Hays DM, Lawrence W, Newton W, Ragab A, Raney B, Soule EH, Sutow WW, Tefft M (1977) Intergroup rhabdomyosarcoma study: preliminary report. Cancer 40: 2015–2026
6. Pinkel D, Pickren J (1961) Rhabdomyosarcoma in children. J Am Med Assoc 175: 293–298
7. Pratt CB, Hustu HO, Fleming ID, Pinkel D (1972) Co-ordinated treatment of childhood rhabdomyosarcoma with surgery, radiotherapy and combination chemotherapy. Cancer Res 32: 606–610
8. Pratt CB, George S (1980) Response of childhood rhabdomyosarcoma (RMS) to combination chemotherapy. Proc Am Assoc Cancer Res (Abstr 723) 21: 181
9. Ransom JL, Pratt CB, Shanks E (1977) Childhood rhabdomyosarcoma of extremity. Results of combined modality therapy. Cancer 40: 2810–2816
10. Tefft M, Fernandez C, Donaldson M, Newton W, Moon TF (1978) Incidence of meningeal involvement by rhabdomyosarcoma of the head and neck in children. Report of Intergroup Rhabdomyosarcoma Study. Cancer 42: 253–258

Benefits and Complications of Combined Management of Children with Malignant Disease

D. Pearson

Department of Radiotherapy and Oncology, Christie Hospital and Holt Radium Institute, Manchester M20 9BX, United Kingdom

Introduction

The modern management of children with malignant diesease requires the close cooperation of the radiotherapist and chemotherapist with surgeons of several disciplines. The clinicians so involved need to be aware of both the benefits and complications which may arise from the combination of the different treatment modalities. Tumours are rare in children; so it is essential that the expertise gathered together for the management of the patients should be in reasonably large oncology centres and also that there is cooperation at both national and international levels to maximise the benefits of treatment.

Benefits

The most important and obvious benefit from the modern management of children's tumours is the improvement in survival rates which has occurred. Table 1 shows this improvement in 3-year survival rates for some of the more common children's tumours. In Hodgkin's disease, embryonal rhabdomyosarcoma, and nephroblastoma this improvement is mainly due to the introduction of cytotoxic chemotherapy, which has been successful both in eliminating micrometastases and in treating metastatic or generalised disease. Its use has also helped to increase the local effectiveness of radiotherapy.
In the brain tumours − namely the astrocytomas and medulloblastomas − improvements in overall survival have been due to different factors. At one time, more than 30% of all children with medulloblastoma died either before or immediately after operation, but by the early 1970s the improvement in neurosurgical techniques, combined with the use of dexamethasone to reduce the intracranial tension considerably reduced this mortality. As a result, survival rates have improved, without any overall change in management, and independent of any effect of cytotoxic drugs.
Not all tumours have this improved survival; an example is neuroblasoma, for which, despite initial good responses to chemotherapy, no maintained improvement in survival rates has been shown.
Other benefits of combined treatment are more difficult to quantify. The controlled clinical trials organised nationally and internationally have certainly increased our knowledge of the natural history of individual tumours and their response to treatment. There is also evidence that children entered into such trials have a better prognosis than those treated in non-patricipating centres.
There is also increasing evidence that the combined use of radiatiotherapy and chemotherapy achieves control of established tumour in more patients than the use of

Table 1. Manchester Children's Tumour Registry: Survival rates at 3 years

	1954–1963 (%)	1964–1968 (%)	1969 and 1970 (%)
Hodgkin's disease	57.7	56.5	66.0
Astrocytoma (cerebellum)	74.1	72.2	85.0
Medulloblastoma	23.1	35.7	66.6
Neuroblastoma	18.0	14.8	27.0
Embryonic sarcoma	23.1	14.8	53.0
Nephroblastoma	25.5	45.0	69.0

radiatiotherapy alone; moreover, a lower dose of radiation is often effective in this type of regime.

This is best illustrated by the management of chest metastases from nephroblastoma. Before the introduction of cytotoxic chemotherapy, about 14% of children with lung metastases were cured using radiation alone at doses of 2,500 cGy in daily fractions over 4 weeks to the whole lung. With actinomycin D and a dose of 1,500 cGy the cure rate was increased to 50%. More recent experience, particularly with rhabdomyosarcoma, does suggest that lower radiation doses can be used to control the primary tumour when combination chemotherapy is given with radiotherapy.

Complications

These can be described as those which may occur during active treatment and those which may occur later, particularly those seen on development of the child.

Immediate Effects

Drug-Radiation Interactions. Interaction between radiation and cytotoxic agents may produce complications. In 1959 D'Angio et al. reported on the enhancement of radiation reactions of the skin when actinomycin D was added to the surgical and radiation treatment of nephroblastoma. Other reactions are also increased, and this can be particularly hazardous when the head and neck region is the site of the primary tumour. An increased degree of mucosal reaction in the larynx and pharynx can be very dangerous in a small child as the congestion and oedema may cause acute airway obstruction.

In addition to these local effects on skin and mucosa, whole organ tolerance may be altered by interaction of radiation and cytotoxic drugs. Toxicity has occurred in liver, lungs and kidneys at lower radiation doses than our previous experience had indicated were tolerable by these organs. Toxic episodes can recur as with recall skin and mucosal reactions, when further courses of the drugs are given; but they become less marked and fade completely as time after radiation increases.

We therefore tried to look at these interactions between drugs and radiation, in the experimental animal. My radiobiology colleagues have looked at various drugs and radiation, in different fractions and at different times. From these experiments which have been described by Pearson et al. (1978) it has been found that the time at which the drug is given in relation to the course of radiation may alter the biological effect. When the drug is given on the same day as the radiation exposure then enhancement occurs, but when the drug is given first and a few days allowed to elapse before irradiation, then there is no enhancement. This confirms our clinical experience, but unfortunately neither the radiobiologist nor the clinician is yet able to determine the best time relationship in order to reduce normal tissue enhancement to a minimum; or, when both are required to be given close together, what reduction in dose levels must be made to prevent organ toxicity.

Opportunistic Infections. The other immediate problem is that infections of all kinds are more likely to occur, because both radiation and chemotherapy are immune depressing treatments. Infections may be much more severe than in normal individuals. Where possible, avoiding exposure, particularly to viral infections, is the best approach. Immune globulins may be used to decrease the severity of any infection that does occur. For other infections continuous surveillance and rapidly introduced treatment is the best that can be offered.

Late Effects

It has been possible to study the late effects of irradiation in childhood because the longest survivors of childhood tumours treated in Manchester have been kept on indefinite follow-up. As yet we do not have as much information about such effects in children treated with combined therapy. Many of the defects which may occur will not manifest themselves for many years, and some certainly will not be apparent until puberty occurs or should occur. I will describe first the late effects of radiation and later what evidence we have for late effects of chemotherapy or combined therapy.

Late Effects of Radiation. Table 2 lists the local effects on skin and soft tissue. It should be stressed that with megavoltage radiation skin scarring and permanent epilation are less likely to occur. However, the thinning of subcutaneous tissue is seen, and as it is also associated with lack of bony development it leads to abnormalities such as thin necks and waists. This can make the buying of clothes quite difficult as these patients are then out of proportion. Abnormalities such as these can cause psychological and social problems and patients may require sympathetic help to accept the situation.

Table 3 shows the skeletal effects which have been recorded. The shortening of the limbs, accompanied by thinning, and the shortening of the spine are understandable and have to be accepted. It should always be possible to avoid scoliosis, by always including the whole width of the spine in the filed of irradiation even if it is only necessary for tumour coverage to go to the midline.

It is important to recognise the complication of the slipped femoral emphysis first described by Chapman et al. in 1980. This occurs in children who have received abdominal or pelvic irradiation and in whom the femoral head had been inadequately shielded. These children complain of pain and a limp, and this should call for an immediate radiograph which will show the displacement of the epiphyses. These can be pinned by an orthopaedic surgeon and the mobility of the hip following this is usually excellent. Considerable problems are likely if these cases are not detected and properly managed.

Exostoses are often asymptomatic and their true incidence is hard to assess as not all children have had x-rays taken of the irradiated area. They should, when detected, be kept

Table 2. Late effects of radiation in children — skin and soft tissue

1)	Scarring ant telangiectasia with high dose radiation
2)	Alopecia
3)	Lack of subcutaneous tissue — thin necks and waists

Table 3. Late effects of radiation in children — skeletal

1)	Lack of growth a) Short spines b) Short limbs c) Asymmetry
2)	Epiphyseal slipping — Femoral
3)	Development of exostoses

Table 4. Late effects of radiation in children — endocrine

1)	*Pituitary and hypothalamus* Growth hormone deficiency
2)	*Gonads* Sterility and failure to develop
3)	*Thyroid* Compensated thyroid dysfunction and hypothyroidism

on regular observation, but if growth occurs or they give rise to symptoms, removal should be undertaken.

Table 4 shows the endocrine effects which have been detected in patients irradiated in childhood. Thyroid dysfunction occurs after neck irradiation both in adults and children. Of the affected children described by Shalet et al. (1977) most showed a raised TSH level, although the T3 and T4 levels remained normal. However, this may proceed to a true biochemical hypothyroidism many years after irradiation; and this can occur quite suddenly after many years of the compensated thyroid dysfunction described. One of the boys showed compensated dysfunction at 14 years and a year later was biochemically hypothyroid, so that it is felt that all these patients should have thyroid function tests performed annually.

A study of long term survivors with brain tumours treated in Manchester (Bamford et al. 1976) showed that many were shorter in stature than expected. In some children this was not explained by their having had spinal irradiation. Endocrine investigations performed and described by Shalet et al. (1976) revealed that these patients had a deficiency of growth hormone. It would seem that a dose of 2,900 cGy in daily fractions over 4 weeks to the pituitary/hypothalamic axis will produce growth hormone deficiency.

Irradiation of the gonads may be expected to produce dysfunction. In girls, when the whole abdomen or pelvis is irradiated, the ovaries are in the primary beam. When the dose exceeds 2,000 cGy, ovarian function is usually destroyed and these girls will require hormone replacement therapy to develop at puberty. In some very young girls however, even at these relatively high doses, development has occurred apparently normally at puberty, and menses appear. One patient became pregnant on two occasions, but for other reasons did not got to term. The foetuses appeared normal. It would appear that some of the ovarian follicles in very young girls may be more resistant to radiation than is the case in older girls.

In boys it is relatively uncommon for the testes to be in the primary beam but if they are, and receive a dose of 3,000 cGy in daily fractions over 4 weeks, then complete testicular failure occurs, and hormone replacement is required at puberty. In most treatments the abominal or pelvic radiation has the lower edge of the field at the symphysis pubis, so that the testis is outside the primary beam. In such patients, normal pubertal development occurs but, as we discovered, sterility is common, often shortly after puberty though it may be delayed for some years. We calculated the likely dose range from the edge of the field to 4 cm below it. The doses ranged from 500–1,000 cGy in 4 weeks and it seems likely that in small boys the testis is usually found at this level. With whole abdominal radiation being less commonly used now in the management of the Wilms' tumour, ovarian and testicular damage is not likely to occur from the radiation.

Second Primary Malignancies. Patients cured of malignancy in childhood may develop second primary neoplasms at a later date. The Late Effects Study Group, as reported by Meadows in a personal communication, has shown that although there is in many patients a genetic predisposition, radiation does increase the risk of a second neoplasm. The group most clearly showing both genetic and radiation effects are the retinoblastoma patients, some of whom develop primary bone tumours at a later date; when radiation has been used in the past, the bone tumour is more likely to occur within the irradiation field. Moreover, the time to the development of the second primary tumour is shorter in this case than when only genetic influences apply.

Late Effects of Combined Treatment. Do radiotherapy and chemotherapy interact to produce worse late effects than either treatment given alone?
The early enhancement of radiation reaction would seem almost certainly to lead to greater scarring and organ loss at a later date. In patients with orbital rhabdomyosarcomas in our study, before we realised that the radiation dose should be reduced, and could probably safely be reduced in combination with chemotherapy, we experienced increased scarring and a more rapid morbidity in the eye. The local damage to the skin and the eye was greater at an earlier time than with radiation alone. Subsequently, when the dose of radiation had been reduced, this effect was not seen.
Radiation and chemotherapy used in the prophylactic treatment of the central nervous system in acute lymphoblastic leukaemia have also been shown to produce late complications. These are listed in Table 5, and have been described by Morris Jones in personal communication. She studied the factors which seemed to be necessary for these effects – a radiation dose greater than 2,000 cGy, intrathecal methotrexate greater than 50 mg/m^2 and systemic methotrexate 40–80 mg/m^2 per week. These effects occur even at this low radiation dose, and at greater frequentcy than is found with higher doses given to children with brain tumours.
Whilst in some children we can avoid radiation damage to gonads, some chemotherapeutic regimes may themselves cause testicular damage. This is seen principally in both children and adults with Hodgkin's disease, but we are beginning to detect gonadal damage in children with brain tumours who received bischlorethyl nitrosourea (BCNU), and this drug given to a fairly high total dose can produce a fatal lung fibrosis.

Will current treatment practices increase the incidence of second malignancies? There may be an increase in reticulo-endothelial second primary malignancies, such as myeloid leukaemia, which is occurring in patients with Hodgkin's disease who have received both radiation and chemotherapy. On the other hand Meadows et al. (1976), reporting a series of patients with Wilms' tumours treated with radiation and actinomycin D, seemed to show a reduction in the incidence of second primaries.

Conclusions

We still have a great deal to achieve in the management of many children's tumours, and we need to continue to search for the best combination of several forms of treatment for any particular tumour. Two aims must be realised:
1. To achieve the highest possible cure rate
2. To reduce to a minimum the complications, both early and late
To achieve this means continued cooperation in management and in the detailed surveillance of the patients indefinitely, so that future late effects can be monitored.

References

1. Bamford FM, Morris Jones PH, Beardwell CG, Ribiero GG, Shalet SM, Pearson D (1976) Residual disabilities in children treated for intra-cranial space-occupying lesions. Cancer 37: 1149–1151
2. Chapman JA, Deakin DP, Green GH (1980) Slipped upper femoral epiphysis after radiotherapy. J Bone Joint Surg 62: 337–339
3. D'Angio GH, Farber S, Maddock CL (1959) Potentiation of x-ray effects by actinomycin D. Radiology 73: 175
4. D'Angio GJ, Meodows A, Miké V, Harris C, Evans A, Jaffe N, Newton W, Schweisguth O, Sutow W, Morris-Jones P (1976) Decreased risk of radiation-associated second malignant neoplasms in actinomycin D treated patients. Cancer (Suppl) 37: 1177–1185
5. Pearson D, Deakin DP, Hendry JH, Moore JV (1978) The interaction of actionomycin D and radiation. Int J Radiat Oncol Biol Phys 4: 71–73
6. Shalet SM, Beardwell CG, Morris Jones PH, Pearson D (1976) The effect of varying doses of cerebral irradiation on growth hormone production in children. Clin Endocrinol 5: 287–290
7. Shalet SM, Rosenstock JD, Beardwell CG, Morris Jones PH, Pearson D (1977) Thyroid dysfunction following external irradiation to the neck for Hodgkin's disease in childhood. Clin Radiol 28: 511–515

Recent Results in Cancer Research

Sponsored by the Swiss League against Cancer. Editor in Chief: P. Rentchnick, Genève